SAFE USES OF CORTISONE

SAFE USES OF CORTISONE

By

WILLIAM McK. JEFFERIES, M.D., F.A.C.P.

Assistant Clinical Professor of Medicine
Case Western Reserve University School of Medicine
Cleveland, Ohio
Consultant in Endocrinology
Euclid Clinic
Lutheran Medical Center
St. Vincent Charity Hospital
University Hospitals of Cleveland

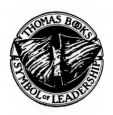

CHARLES C THOMAS · PUBLISHER
Springfield · Illinois · U.S.A.

Published and Distributed Throughout the World by
CHARLES C THOMAS • PUBLISHER
2600 South First Street
Springfield, Illinois 62717 U.S.A.

©*1981, by* CHARLES C THOMAS • PUBLISHER

ISBN 0-398-04531-3

Library of Congress Catalog Card Number: 81-5823

*With THOMAS BOOKS careful attention is given to all details of
manufacturing and design. It is the Publisher's desire to present books that are
satisfactory as to their physical qualities and artistic possibilities and
appropriate for their particular use. THOMAS BOOKS will be true to those
laws of quality that assure a good name and good will.*

Library of Congress Cataloging in Publication Data

Jefferies, William McK.
  Safe uses of cortisone.

  Includes bibliographical references and index.
  1. Cortisone — Therapeutic use. 2. Cortisone —
Physiological effect. I. Title. [DNLM: 1. Cortisone —
Therapeutic use. 2. Hydrocortisone — Therapeutic use.
WK 755 J45s]
RM292.4.C67J43   615'.364   81-5823
ISBN 0-398-04531-3   AACR2

Printed in the United States of America
C-1

PREFACE

THE POTENTIAL of cortisone and hydrocortisone in clinical medicine has been confused by numerous factors. When agents that initially were thought to provide one of the greatest advances in therapy in the history of medicine were found to be capable of causing numerous serious and sometimes catastrophic side effects, both physicians and patients understandably reacted with alarm. Unfortunately, the reaction was so great that perspective has been lost. Furthermore, misunderstanding has resulted from failure to differentiate between physiologic and pharmacologic dosages and effects, from confusion of natural steroids with more potent derivatives, from a lack of knowledge of the nature of beneficial effects, and from other, more subtle factors.

Cortisone and hydrocortisone are natural hormones and, when properly administered, are as safe as any other naturally produced hormones. In addition to its primary role in response to stress of any type, hydrocortisone has beneficial symptomatic effects in many diseases of humans, but its use has been limited because of fear of the harmful side effects that may occur with the pharmacologic dosages that have been customary.

With a thirty-year background of experience with clinical uses of cortisone and hydrocortisone, the author reviews the cortisone story from its beginnings and presents an optimum program of administration of safe, physiologic dosages in adrenal insufficiency and congenital adrenal hyperplasia. Employment of safe dosages on a proper schedule has demonstrated a promising potential in patients with gonadal dysfunction with or without infertility, rheumatoid arthritis, allergic rhinitis, asthma, recently recognized autoimmune disorders such as hyperthyroidism with diffuse goiter, chronic thyroiditis, and diabetes mellitus, and common clinical problems such as functional hypoglycemia, hirsutism, acne, and chronic cystic mastitis.

v

The relative frequency and clinical significance of low adrenal reserve as a cause for unexplained chronic fatigue or functional hypoglycemia and as a possible contributing factor in many allergies provides another area of therapeutic promise. Recent evidence regarding the mechanisms of physiologic effects of hydrocortisone are discussed in relation to these areas of clinical potential.

INTRODUCTION

THE ADRENALS are a major component of the body's defense against stress, and this includes any type of injury or infection. The malaise associated with any severe injury or illness can be alleviated by the administration of suitable doses of adrenocortical hormone. It is apparent that the secretion of a gland that has such remarkable potential may affect the body's reaction to any unpleasant condition, whether physical or psychological, injury or disease. Hydrocortisone is the most important of the hormones produced by the adrenal cortex. Cortisone is converted to hydrocortisone after absorption, hence its effects are qualitatively the same. Unfortunately, when cortisone was first introduced to clinical medicine, the amount of this hormone that was normally produced by human subjects was not known, nor was an optimum route or schedule of administration. Furthermore, under some circumstances the administration of a large dosage of either cortisone or hydrocortisone might be dramatically beneficial; under others, the same dosage might cause great harm. This combination of properties has resulted in much confusion regarding the therapeutic usefulness versus toxic potential of these steroids in clinical medicine.

While I was a student and house officer at the Massachusetts General Hospital, 1939 to 1942, I was fortunate to have Dr. Fuller Albright as an instructor. Dr. Albright was a pioneer investigator of the function of the adrenal cortex in humans, and he stimulated my interest in the relationships of the adrenals and other endocrine glands to stress. During World War II, while serving as a flight surgeon in India, Burma, and China for two and a half years, I had an opportunity to observe the effects of intense psychological and physical stress on airmen.[1] Subsequently, I spent two years on a research fellowship with the Thyroid Clinic at the Massachusetts General Hospital under Dr.

James Howard Means and a year with the Endocrine Clinic under Dr. Albright.

In early 1949 Dr. Albright received a small supply of Compound F, the adrenocortical steroid that was later to be called hydrocortisone or cortisol, for clinical studies. Dr. Philip Hench and his associates at the Mayo Clinic had recently reported impressive beneficial effects of cortisone acetate and adrenocorticotrophic hormone (ACTH) in patients with arthritis,[2] and Dr. Albright decided to determine the effects of Compound F upon metabolic balances in a human subject. Drs. Paul Fourman and Frederick Bartter collaborated with him in the study.[3]

Meanwhile, I had been invited to take charge of the Endocrine Clinic and Endocrine Research Laboratory at University Hospitals in Cleveland, Ohio. Shortly after my arrival in the summer of 1949 I received a supply of cortisone acetate from Dr. Elmer Alpert of Merck, Sharp and Dohme, Inc. and of adrenocorticotropic hormone (ACTH) from Dr. John Mote of the Armour Laboratories to use for clinical investigation. Later the Upjohn Company provided a generous supply of cortisone acetate and hydrocortisone for clinical studies. When cortisone acetate and hydrocortisone became available for general clinical use in 1950, I was delegated to see every patient given either of these agents at University Hospitals for over a year, and most of such patients subsequently. This experience provided a perspective of the beneficial and the harmful effects of the clinical uses of these agents, and in 1955 I summarized the current status of their use in clinical medicine.[4]

At this time I became intrigued with the beneficial effects of small doses of cortisone or hydrocortisone in women with ovarian dysfunction and infertility. As a result of my previous experience with the duration of effects of hydrocortisone and with the treatment of patients with spontaneous adrenal insufficiency (Addison's disease), I had patients divide the daily dosage so that a portion was taken before each meal and at bedtime. The results of this work were published, but patents on cortisone acetate and hydrocortisone were terminating, and the medical profession and general public had become disenchanted with these agents because of the toxic effects that occurred with larger dosages.

As I continued clinical studies with safe, physiologic dosages of cortisone acetate and hydrocortisone, interesting potential uses were encountered that were either new or had been forgotten. I continued to present at meetings and publish results of our work, and following each presentation a number of interested inquiries were received, but nothing more happened. In retrospect it appears that the failure of pharmaceutical houses to follow up promotionally in the manner that physicians are accustomed to expecting when improvements in therapy are reported caused interested physicians to decide that the therapy must not have been as effective as my reports implied. There have, however, been no reports indicating that any results I have published could not be substantiated.

As time passed, the attitude of grant committees and editorial boards changed. Requests for funds to study these new uses were denied, and reports of the promising potential of the safe dosages were turned down for publication. It became evident that cortisone and hydrocortisone had achieved such a bad reputation that many members of these committees or boards hesitated to accept or publish any report that suggested they might have further potential benefit.

In the course of my researches I was in touch with Fuller Albright until his death and also with Dwight Ingle, the distinguished physiologist at the University of Chicago School of Medicine. Both offered encouragement. I saw Dwight each year at the Laurentian Hormone Conference, where we had lively discussions of our mutual interests in adrenal physiology. He had a continuing interest in my observations on patients and encouraged my attempts to have these published. Unfortunately, he died of a heart attack on July 28, 1978.

Many of the investigators who participated in the first clinical studies with these steroids have retired or died, and younger investigators have been so strongly indoctrinated with the hazards of glucocorticoids that they seem to be unaware of the safety of physiologic dosages, so I decided to review the cortisone story in an attempt to restore perspective and to present my observations with the hope of stimulating others to return to the study of the *physiologic* effects of hydrocortisone and its proper place in clinical medicine.

One of the aspects of this type of therapy that has strained its credibility is the wide variety of pathologic disorders that are benefited. It is difficult to believe that one therapeutic agent could help so many conditions. Yet, recent findings regarding the etiologic role of autoimmunity in many diseases whose cause was unknown provide an explanation of some of these previously unexplained beneficial effects, since, for reasons that are not clear, glucocorticoids are known to benefit autoimmune disorders. In fact, the mechanism of any of the beneficial effects of glucocorticoids is not known. Speculations regarding recent studies in this area provide further reasons for encouraging continuing investigations in this field. Evidence that physiologic dosages of cortisone or hydrocortisone may improve resistance to viral infections, in contrast to the known harmful effects of pharmacologic dosages that decrease such resistance, opens another area warranting careful study.

Many of the promising clinical uses described in this book require further investigation to determine the proper scope of such uses, and additional experience is advisable to confirm the safety of this therapy in the hands of others, but in over one thousand patient years of experience with the dosages described, none of the harmful potential of larger, *pharmacologic* dosages has been encountered. It would have been easier to relax and forget the cortisone problem, but the therapeutic promise of this type of treatment is too great.

In writing this book no attempt has been made to refer to the entire literature regarding the various subjects discussed — it is much too vast — but an attempt has been made to cite pertinent reports; from these the interested reader may obtain a more complete bibliography on a particular subject. Much of the book consists of case reports because these represent experiments of nature, and careful observations often provide evidence of clinical efficacy and clues to further advances in knowledge in a manner that is not possible in statistical analyses or double-blind placebo studies.

If this book stimulates researchers and clinicians to reevaluate their fears about the hazards of cortisone therapy and causes them to consider further possible beneficial effects of physiologic dosages, its purpose will have been achieved.

REFERENCES

1. Jefferies WMcK: Stress in personnel flying the "Hump." *Bull U.S. Army Med Dept 6:*603-610, Nov., 1946.
2. Hench PS, Kendall EC, Slocumb CH, and Polley HF: The effect of a hormone of the adrenal cortex (17-hydroxy-11-dehydrocorticosterone: Compound E) and of pituitary adrenocorticotropic hormone on rheumatoid arthritis: preliminary report. *Proc Staff Meet Mayo Clin 24:*181-197, 1949.
3. Fourman P, Bartter FC, Albright F, Dempsey EL, Carroll E, Alexander J: Effects of 17 hydroxy-corticosterone (Compound F) in man. *J Clin Invest 29:*1462-1473, 1950.
4. Jefferies WMcK: The present status of ACTH, cortisone and related steroids in clinical medicine. *N Engl J Med 253:*441-446, 1955.

ACKNOWLEDGMENTS

I AM INDEBTED to Dr. George W. Thorn and to Dr. Sibley Hoobler for reviewing the manuscript and making helpful suggestions; to the Brush Foundation of Cleveland and the Euclid Clinic Research Foundation for providing funds for most of my clinical research; to Dr. David R. Weir, Mr. Tommy McCuistion, and Mr. Robert Cheshire for encouragement and counsel; to my nurse, Mrs. Carol Ankuda, for assistance in collecting and recording patient data; to technicians Jeanne Wynne and Cheryl Hach for their assistance in collecting and recording data as well as for their meticulous laboratory work; to Mrs. Janet Parodi for assistance in organizing data and typing most of the manuscript; to Mrs. Margaret Henning for assisting in library research and reviewing the manuscript; and to the numerous other technicians, secretaries, research fellows and patients who have participated in these studies. Special thanks should also go to the Armour Laboratories for contributing ACTH and to Merck, Sharp and Dohme and the Upjohn Company for contributing cortisone acetate and hydrocortisone for use in many of these studies.

CONTENTS

SAFE USES OF CORTISONE

Chapter 1

BACKGROUND

Iɴ 1949 when Dr. Philip Hench and his associates at the Mayo Clinic reported the remarkable effects of cortisone and adrenocorticotropic hormone (ACTH) on patients with rheumatoid arthritis,[1] their discovery was greeted as a major advance in the field of medicine. The Nobel Prize awarded for this work reflected the significance that was attached to it. Not only were patients previously crippled with arthritis helped to get back on their feet and become active members of society again, but patients with other so-called "collagen diseases" such as disseminated lupus erythematosus, polyarteritis nodosa, and scleroderma were dramatically benefited; patients with allergies such as bronchial asthma, hay fever, and eczema received impressive relief; patients with some types of leukemia and other malignancies went into temporary remissions; and those with numerous other disorders experienced unprecedented improvement from these agents. It is not surprising that cortisone came to be known as the "miracle medicine." Yet, within a few years, cortisone fell into such disfavor that it was considered a dangerous drug whose use should be reserved for serious illnesses when no other treatment was effective. That it is a normal hormone was largely forgotten, and that many patients take it for years with no harmful side effects was generally overlooked. Actually, many patients cannot live normal lives without it, and while taking it they are as normal as any healthy person. Furthermore, there are other potential uses of this medication in safe dosages that appear even more promising than the known uses of the hazardous dosages. There is even convincing evidence that it can improve resistance to the common cold and influenza!

How could such a situation occur? What is the evidence that cortisone can be safe? In what other conditions does it show therapeutic potential? Why is it still one of the most promising

3

therapeutic agents of all time? As an initial step in attempting to answer these questions, the history of the cortisone story will be briefly reviewed and an effort made to restore perspective.

HISTORY

In 1929 Dr. Hench saw a patient whose rheumatoid arthritis had "disappeared" within a week after the sudden development of jaundice.[2] Later he noted that pregnancy often resulted in impressive improvement of arthritis, followed by a relapse after delivery.[3] Subsequently, temporary improvement in rheumatoid arthritis was noted when patients underwent such varied clinical conditions as surgical procedures, general anesthesia without surgery, therapy with ergosterol, estrogens, or testosterone, a high fat (ketogenic) diet, or starvation.[4] After much speculation and clinical investigation, he decided that the agent responsible for improvement under these numerous apparently unrelated circumstances might be a normal adrenocortical hormone.

In 1930 Dr. Edward C. Kendall had undertaken a chemical and physiologic investigation of the adrenal cortex in the biochemical laboratories of the Mayo Foundation for Medical Education and Research.[5] In 1934 the first crystalline compounds were separated and designated "Compounds A, B, C, and D." In the following year Compounds E and F were isolated, and chemical formulas were assigned to these compounds in 1937 and 1938. Dr. Dwight Ingle, who was working in Dr. Kendall's laboratory, demonstrated that Compound E had a beneficial effect on muscular work capacity in rats.[6] Later this compound was found to influence carbohydrate metabolism, and other investigators showed that it increased physiologic resistance to stress or cold and to toxic substances such as typhoid vaccine.[7]

By 1940 it had become evident that investigation of the effects of Compounds A, B, E, and F in human subjects was desirable, but no method of obtaining sufficient supplies for clinical studies was known. In the fall of 1941, just before Pearl Harbor, requests were made to the National Research Council by the medical departments of the Army and Navy for a large supply of the hormones of the adrenal cortex, because it was believed that they might be of value in the event of military conflict. Interest in these hormones was heightened by a rumor that pilots of the German Luftwaffe were injected with adrenal cortical extract and that this enabled them to fly with ease at altitudes of 40,000 feet or more.[5] During the war twenty-two laboratories in the United States were attempting to prepare hormones of the adrenal cortex, but by 1945, after interest in potential military use of adrenocortical hormones had subsided, only the laboratories of the Mayo Foundation and of Merck & Co., Inc. persisted in this search.

The combined efforts of these two laboratories resulted in the production of a sufficient quantity of Compound E to initiate limited clinical studies in the spring of 1948. Dr. Randall Sprague and his associates received a small quantity for treatment of three patients with adrenal insufficiency at the Mayo Clinic, and they tried dosages of 50 and 100 mg intramuscularly daily with beneficial effects.[8] In September, 1948, when Hench and his group received a supply of Compound E for clinical investigation in arthritics, the larger dosage of 100 mg daily was decided upon.[1] In retrospect, this was a fortuitous decision because, with the preparation and schedule of administration they used, a smaller dosage might not have produced impressive clinical benefit.

The first arthritic patient to be given Compound E was a twenty-nine year old woman with severe rheumatoid arthritis of four and one-half years duration who had received many treatments without significant improvement. On September 21, 1948, she received her first injection of 50 mg of Compound E intramuscularly, and this was continued twice daily. The following day little evidence of improvement was apparent, but when she awoke on September 23 she noted much less muscular soreness. On September 24 painful morning stiffness was entirely gone, and whereas she had scarcely been able to walk three days previously, she now walked with only a slight limp. By the seventh day of treatment, "articular as well as muscular stiffness had almost completely disappeared, and tenderness, pain on motion, and even swellings, had markedly lessened."[1]

Over the next six months a total of fourteen patients with severe or moderately severe rheumatoid arthritis were treated. Between September, 1948,. and January, 1949, Compound E was used, but it was then found that the less expensive and more easily prepared Compound E acetate "was absorbed with sufficient promptness," so subsequently patients received this preparation. An interesting comment was that "early preparations used for our first three patients were potent and devoid of side effects," but then difficulties were encountered. When two subsequent preparations were substituted in patients who had previously been benefited by injections of Compound E, articular flare-ups promptly occurred, and sedimentation rates rose quickly. It was noted that in earlier preparations crystals were fairly large, possibly slowing absorption and providing a longer sustained effect, whereas later preparations contained smaller crystals, easier to administer and more rapidly absorbed.

Because larger doses of the new preparations seemed necessary to produce rapid clinical improvement, and because 100 mg of Compound E acetate was the chemical equivalent of 89 mg of Compound E, Hench and his group were inclined to attribute the requirement for larger doses to the change to the E acetate. They accordingly began to administer 300 mg Compound E acetate on the first day, followed by 100 mg daily thereafter,[9, 10] still on a schedule of one or two intramuscular injections daily.

In retrospect it seems likely that some of the difference in therapeutic effectiveness could have been related to the difference in crystal size, the larger, more slowly absorbed crystals providing a greater antiarthritic effect than the smaller, more rapidly absorbed ones, especially with the schedule of administration of only once or twice daily that was used. At the time, however, this possibility was apparently not considered.

After patients obtained initial optimum improvement, generally within seven to fourteen days, their daily dosage was reduced to 75, 50, or even 25 mg, with the hope of finding a smaller, more economical, effective maintenance level. Unfortunately, flare-ups occurred and sedimentation rates rose promptly in most cases treated in this manner. They therefore concluded that "so far a minimum daily dosage of 75 mg to 100 mg seems required and sometimes such a dose does not entirely control symptoms and sedimentation rates." They mentioned cushingoid changes in only one of their patients, the first whom they treated and the one who seemed to be particularly resistant to treatment, requiring repeated administration of larger doses. Later, signs of hypercortisonism began to appear in other patients, so Compound E acetate therapy was interrupted, with intervals of several days to weeks between courses. They stated,

> . . . we observed no notable reactions of toxicity when later preparations of Compound E or E acetate were used. Transient epigastric pain occurred occasionally but was relieved with cessation of dosage for a few days. Transient edema, generally pretibial, occurred occasionally, but it disappeared, sometimes spontaneously, or when the dosage was reduced.[10]

The term "cortisone" was not introduced until several months after the initial report.[9] Because corticosterone, Kendall's Compound B, was one of the first adrenocortical steroids to be identified, other adrenocortical steroids were often termed as chemical relatives of this steroid. Hence Compound E was also known as 11-dehydro-17-hydroxy-corticosterone. The term cortisone was introduced as a simplification of the unwieldy chemical name for practicing physicians and the general public. Later, when Kendall's Compound F was found to be equally effective in the treatment of arthritis, it came to be called "hydrocortisone" because it differed from cortisone only in the presence of a hydroxyl group instead of a ketone group on the eleventh carbon atom. Subsequently, chemists recommended that hydrocortisone be termed cortisol because the suffix -one referred to a ketone grouping, such as was present in cortisone, but the proper suffix for a hydroxyl group was -ol. Unfortunately, the spoken words cortisol and cortisone sound so similar that they may be confused, so many clinicians have continued to refer to Compound F as hydrocortisone, except when referring to its level in the blood, when the term "plasma cortisol" is more commonly used. Because hydrocortisone is the chief glucocorticoid produced normally by the human adrenal cortex, cortisone being converted to it prior to the production of effects in the tissues, it is more frequently used for physiologic effects today.

In retrospect, besides the interrupted courses, there are other possible explanations of why so few side effects were observed in these initial studies. It is now known that under normal, unstressed conditions the adrenals produce the equivalent of 35 to 40 mg of cortisone acetate taken by mouth in divided doses daily,[11] so the initial dosages used by Hench and his group were considerably in excess of this normal production and, hence, would be expected to produce the characteristic effects of hypercortisonism. Because these dosages were administered intramuscularly in preparations that were relatively rapidly absorbed, however, and in only one or two injections daily, and since it has been demonstrated that the same total daily dosage of hydrocortisone taken in four divided doses before meals and at bedtime is more effective than when taken in two divided doses at twelve-hour intervals,[12] the schedule of the early injections would be less effective and less likely to produce side effects than the same total dosage being administered at more frequent intervals throughout the twenty-four hours.

Hence, if the first preparation used by Hench had been the type of cortisone acetate that is available today, and if it had been administered in divided dosages as it is today, a daily dosage of 100 mg would probably have produced more side effects more quickly, and smaller dosages might have been clinically effective. *It should, therefore, be borne in mind that conclusions regarding dosages necessary for clinical effects based upon the observations of the earlier investigators may not be valid when applied to later preparations and schedules of therapy.*

In addition, it is now known that smaller dosages of cortisone may take ten to fourteen days to produce impressive improvement in arthritis so that possible beneficial effects of smaller dosages used as initial therapy might have been missed because they were not continued for a sufficient period of time, even if they had been administered on an optimum schedule.

After it was found that cortisone acetate and hydrocortisone were effective by mouth[13, 14] when the daily dosage was divided into several portions, beneficial effects in numerous diseases were reported. These were summarized in an excellent review by Thorn and his associates.[15] Unfortunately, reports of undesirable side effects also began to multiply. These included rounded or "moon face," thinning of the skin with easy bruisability and appearance of striae, subcutaneous hemorrhages, osteoporosis, spontaneous fractures, peptic ulcers, and fluid retention with edema. Initial dosages were, therefore, reduced to 100 mg daily and maintenance dosages to 50 mg daily, and the undesirable side effects did not appear quite so quickly, but they still occurred. Later, two even more alarming side effects became evident. Patients on cortisone therapy demonstrated a diminished resistance to infection, and if they underwent even minor surgical procedures, they might collapse and die under the anesthetic.

Such complications understandably caused alarm and consternation on the part of the medical profession and the public. A therapeutic agent that had been welcomed as a miraculous advance had been found to be potentially a treacherous poison. Derivatives of cortisone and hydrocortisone that had greater anti-inflammatory and less sodium-retaining effects, such as prednisone, prednisolone, triamcinolone, methyl prednisolone, and dexamethasone, were introduced with the hope that they would be safer, but the only side effect that was reduced was the sodium-retaining effect, and the other hazardous potentials remained. This group of steroids, which had in common the property of stimulating the conversion of protein to carbohydrate (gluconeogenesis), came to be termed glucocorticoids.

Reports of additional serious and sometimes devastating complications of glucocorticoid therapy began to multiply; ophthalmologists reported development of cataracts and aggravation of glaucoma; internists and general practitioners reported osteoporosis with pathologic fractures, development of peptic ulcers with occasional perforation, lowering of resistance to infection, development of diabetes mellitus, and appearance of serious psychological disorders and even psychoses. Surgeons reported possible interference with wound healing as well as collapse and death after general anesthetic for relatively minor surgery.

Not every patient treated with glucocorticoids developed such alarming complications, but some did, and practically every practitioner encountered one or more serious complications of this type. It is not surprising that the attitude of physicians toward glucocorticoid therapy reversed from enthusiasm to alarm and that reports advocating reservation of the therapeutic use of these agents for serious, life-threatening diseases for which no other therapy was effective replaced the widespread enthusiastic use for many diseases that had previously been prevalent. Medical literature was swamped with reports of grim complications of glucocorticoid therapy, optimism gave way to pessimism, and a situation gradually developed in which perspective was lost.

Any dosage of any glucocorticoid was considered potentially hazardous. Reports of undesirable effects often failed to state the dosage and duration of administration, implying that all dosages were capable of producing similar effects. The term "cortisone therapy" was applied indiscriminately to treatment with other glucocorticoids, making it difficult to evaluate differences between glucocorticoid preparations or even to determine what steroid a patient had received. The literature abounded with statements that all glucocorticoid therapy is dangerous, hence it should not be started except as a last resort and should be discontinued as soon as possible. For over twenty years physicians have been indoctrinated with this concept.

REFERENCES

1. Hench PS, Kendall EC, Slocumb CH, Polley HF: The effect of a hormone of the adrenal cortex (17-hydroxy-11-dehydrocorticosterone: Compound E) and of pituitary adrenocorticotropic hormone on rheumatoid arthritis; preliminary report. *Proc Staff Meet Mayo Clin, 24:*181-197, 1949.
2. Hench PS: Analgesia accompanying hepatitis and jaundice in cases of chronic arthritis, fibrositis and sciatic pain. *Proc Staff Meet Mayo Clin 8:*430-436, 1933.
3. Hench PS: The ameliorating effect of pregnancy on chronic atrophic (infectious, rheumatoid) arthritis, fibrositis and intermittent hydrarthrosis. *Proc Staff Meet Mayo Clin 13:*161-167, 1938.
4. Polley HF, Slocumb CH: Behind the scenes with cortisone and ACTH. *Mayo Clin Proc 51:*471-477, 1976.
5. Kendall EC: Some observations on the hormone of the adrenal cortex designated Compound E. *Proc Staff Meet Mayo Clin 24:*298-301, 1949.

6. Ingle, DJ: Work capacity of the adrenalectomized rat treated with cortin. *Am J Physiol 116:*622-625, 1936.

7. Kendall EC: Adrenal Cortex. *Arch Pathol 32:*474-501, 1941.

8. Sprague RG, Power MH, Mason HL, Claxton HE: Metabolic effects of synthetic Compound E (17-hydroxy-11-dehydrocorticosterone) in two patients with Addison's disease and one with coexisting Addison's disease and diabetes mellitus (Abstract). *J Clin Invest 28:*812, 1949.

9. Sprague RG, Power MH, Mason HL, Albert A, Mathieson DR, Hench PS, Kendall EC, Slocumb CH, Polley HF: Observations on the physiologic effects of cortisone and ACTH in man. *Arch Intern Med 85:*199-258, 1950.

10. Hench PS, Kendall EC, Slocumb, CH, Polley HF: Effects of cortisone acetate and pituitary ACTH on rheumatoid arthritis, rheumatic fever and certain other conditions. *Arch Intern Med 85:*545-666, 1950.

11. Jefferies WMcK: Low dosage glucocorticoid therapy. *Arch Intern Med 119:*265-278, 1967.

12. Jefferies WMcK: Glucocorticoids and Ovulation. In Greenblatt RB (Ed.): *Ovulation.* Philadelphia, Lippincott, 1966, pp. 62-74.

13. Freyberg RH, Traeger CH, Adams CH, Kuscu T, Wainerdi H, Bonomo I: Effectiveness of cortisone administered orally. *Science 112:*429, 1950.

14. Ward LE, Slocumb CH, Polley HF, Lowman EW, Hench PS: Clinical effects of cortisone administered orally to patients with rheumatoid arthritis. *Proc Staff Meet Mayo Clin 26:*361-370, 1951.

15. Thorn GW, Jenkins D, Laidlaw JC, Goetz FC, Dingman JF, Arons WL, Streeten DHP, McCracken BH: Pharmacologic aspects of adrenocortical steroids and ACTH in man. *N Engl J Med 248:*232-245, 284-294, 323-337, 369-378, 414-423, 588-601, 632-646, 1953.

Chapter 2

SOURCES OF CONFUSION

THAT CORTISONE and hydrocortisone are normal hormones of the adrenal cortex implies that in physiologic dosages they must be safe. This implication is confirmed by the clinical experience of patients with adrenal insufficiency or congenital adrenal hyperplasia. When given suitable maintenance dosages, they can take cortisone or hydrocortisone indefinitely without undesirable side effects and enjoy perfectly normal health. Other patients in our clinics have received small, physiologic dosages of cortisone or hydrocortisone for various conditions that will be described later, totalling *over one thousand patient years of experience*. Other than an occasional incidence of acid indigestion, usually resulting from taking the steroid on an empty stomach, or a rare instance of a patient being allergic to an ingredient of the filler in the steroid tablet, no undesirable side effects whatsoever have occurred.

It is not generally realized that the dangerous side effects of glucocorticoid therapy occur only with certain dosages and not with others. That there is a tremendous difference between the effects of small "physiologic" dosages and those of larger "pharmacologic" dosages has not been emphasized.

For example, it is widely recognized that glucocorticoids, including cortisone and hydrocortisone, produce a negative nitrogen balance, but this is not a normal physiologic effect. If it were, all hypoadrenal patients on replacement therapy would be in negative nitrogen balance, but they obviously are not. Ingle and Baker[1] in 1953 emphasized that cortisone and hydrocortisone inhibit anabolism only when administered in excess, but this fact apparently received little attention. The few metabolic balance studies that have been performed on patients with adrenal insufficiency clearly demonstrate that physiologic replacement dosages do not cause nitrogen loss.[2, 3] Recent studies in rats have shown that corticosterone administration does not

12

cause protein loss and cessation of growth until dosages sufficient to raise plasma levels of steroid above the normal range are administered.[4] The concept that a negative nitrogen balance is a normal physiologic effect of cortisone or hydrocortisone is therefore as erroneous as one that hypoglycemia is a normal physiologic effect of insulin.

When applied to hormone actions a "physiologic" dosage implies one that promotes normal function whereas a "pharmacologic" dosage is one in excess of normal requirements and, hence, one that might alter normal function. To determine the normal physiologic effects of any hormone, it must be administered to subjects deficient in this hormone and in no other and in a dosage comparable to the level of production of this hormone in normal subjects. Unfortunately, few studies of the effects of cortisone or hydrocortisone have been made under such circumstances.

Because the beneficial therapeutic effects in rheumatoid arthritis and other diseases were obtained with dosages of 50-150 mg daily, metabolic balance studies and other clinical investigations of their effects employed comparable dosages.[2, 5-20] It is not surprising, therefore, that physicians became familiar with the pharmacologic, rather than the physiologic, effects of these steroids. In a few studies,[2, 3, 7] dosages of cortisone acetate of 50 mg or less per day were administered to patients with adrenal insufficiency, but these observations were either incidental to studies of effects of other steroids or the manner of administration was different from that employed clinically today.

All other studies of the metabolic effects of these steroids have involved the administration of dosages in excess of normal requirements and in most cases to subjects who have not had adrenal insufficiency. The well-known effects of glucocorticoids are, therefore, not their normal physiologic ones but those resulting from administering excessive doses to subjects, many of whom did not need them. These "pharmacologic" effects include excessive sodium and fluid retention, potassium depletion, nitrogen and calcium loss, and elevation of blood sugar.

The failure to differentiate between physiologic and pharmacologic effects has been a major factor in the confusion regarding the clinical value of these agents. When it was found that a normal replacement dosage for an adrenalectomized patient was 35-40 mg of cortisone acetate or hydrocortisone daily, it became evident that dosages above this level were in excess of physiologic requirements, but by this time such serious side effects of the larger dosages had been reported that cortisone and hydrocortisone had achieved a reputation of being dangerous drugs. The possibility that smaller dosages might be safe was not considered, and patients receiving any dosage were thought to be in jeopardy.

With cortisone or hydrocortisone, as with any normal hormone, there are three dosage ranges that can be administered:

1. *Replacement dosage.* In the case of hydrocortisone, this is a dosage equal to that which, in association with physiologic amounts of sodium-retaining and androgenic steroids, is necessary to maintain a totally adrenalectomized patient in normal health in the unstressed state. Physiologic studies indicate that the average daily production of hydrocortisone by human adrenals under basal conditions is approximately 15-20 mg, but this dosage will not maintain a totally adrenalectomized patient. Studies with cortisone acetate in four doses daily (with meals and at bedtime) indicate that approximately 35-40 mg daily is necessary to inhibit endogenous adrenal steroid production to zero,[21] and this dosage will satisfactorily maintain an adrenalectomized patient with a minimum of supplementary sodium-retaining steroid. Hence, this may be considered a *replacement dosage.* Because hydrocortisone is slightly more potent than cortisone acetate, a replacement dosage of hydrocortisone is approximately 32-35 mg daily. The discrepancy between the 20 mg average daily production by normal adrenals and the 32-36 mg necessary to suppress normal adrenocortical activity implies that, when taken by mouth in tablet form, even in divided doses, cortisone acetate or hydrocortisone is only approximately 60 percent as efficient as when the hormone is naturally produced by the adrenals and released directly into the blood in accordance with bodily needs.

If a replacement dosage is given to a patient with intact adrenals, it will, therefore, suppress his or her adrenal function completely, but because the ultimate effect is a level of glucocorticoid not in excess of normal requirements, the effects of hypercortisonism will not develop. If the suppression of endogenous adrenal function persists sufficiently long, the subject may not be able to respond adequately to stress, and he or she may experience temporary adrenal insufficiency after glucocorticoid therapy is withdrawn.

2. *Suprareplacement dosages.* These are in excess of normal physiologic requirements. In the case of cortisone or hydrocortisone, these would be dosages larger than 40 mg daily. These are the dosages implied in most clinical literature, and if continued for a sufficient period of time they can produce all of the undesirable side effects of hypercortisonism.

3. *Subreplacement dosages.* These are dosages less than normal replacement dosages and, hence, are capable of suppressing endogenous adrenal function only partly. It has been demonstrated that when subjects with intact adrenals receive less than full replacement dosages of cortisone acetate or hydrocortisone, endogenous adrenal function is suppressed only sufficiently to achieve a normal total glucocorticoid level.[21] For example, subjects receiving 20 mg (5 mg four times) daily of cortisone acetate have their endogenous adrenal steroid production decreased by approximately 60 percent, and subjects receiving 10 mg (2.5 mg four times) daily have their adrenal steroid production decreased by approximately 30 percent (Fig. 1). The residual functioning tissue is adequate for normal response to stresses such as respiratory or gastrointestinal infections or major surgery.[21] This is not surprising in view of the great functional reserve of the adrenals as documented by the evidence reported by Barker[22] that adrenal insufficiency in the unstressed state does not occur unless 90 percent or more of the cortical tissue is destroyed. Hence, subjects receiving subreplacement dosages of 5 mg or less four times daily have neither hypercortisonism nor significant impairment of resistance to stress.

Although it is theoretically possible that ability to respond to overwhelming stress might be diminished, the ability to tolerate major surgical procedures without supplementary steroid indicates that such impairment is not sufficient to be a clinical prob-

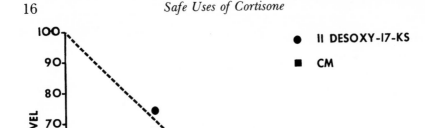

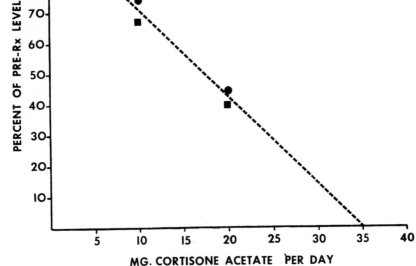

Figure 1. Effects of low dosages of cortisone acetate upon urinary excretion of 11-desoxy-17-KS and hydrocortisone (cortisol) metabolites (CM) from endogenous sources. From William McK Jefferies, Low Dosage Glucocorticoid Therapy, *Archives of Internal Medicine, 119:*265-278. Copyright 1967, the American Medical Association. Reprinted by permission.

lem. Such subreplacement dosages not only leave a sufficient amount of functioning adrenal tissue to enable response to stress but also avoid the complete suppression of endogenous androgen production that probably causes a higher incidence of undesirable side effects with larger doses in women than in men. Many patients who need subreplacement dosages have low adrenal reserve, so the administration of such dosages actually improves the adrenals' ability to respond to stress in these cases.

The schedule of administering cortisone acetate or hydrocortisone every eight hours or four times daily is followed because of evidence that normal blood levels and some metabolic effects of a single dose of hydrocortisone do not last longer than eight hours.[23] For practical purposes, dividing the total daily dosage into four parts taken before each meal and at bedtime has two advantages. It is easier for a patient to remember to take a medication at these times than at other times, hence this schedule provides a convenient way of spreading out the day's dosage. Furthermore, when glucocorticoids are taken just before meals, the ingestion of food tends to counteract the tendency to develop acid indigestion from the stimulation of gastric acid and pepsin produced by the steroid. For the bedtime dose, patients are instructed to drink milk or take an antacid with the medication.

The schedule on which the daily dosage is administered is apparently important not only in the achievement of clinical benefit but also in the avoidance of undesirable side effects. In our studies, administration of cortisone acetate or of hydrocortisone in doses of 5 mg four times daily produced no elevation of plasma 17-hydroxycorticosteroids (17-OHST), nor of excretion of urinary 17-OHST, nor any metabolic changes characteristic of glucocorticoid excess[21] (Fig. 2). After initiation of cortisone or hydrocortisone therapy at this dosage, up to 10 days are required before a new stable state is reached.

Shuster and Williams[24] have reported that a single dose of cortisone acetate as small as 12.5 mg daily administered to normal subjects caused increased excretion of 17-OHST. Their data indicate that urine collections for 17-OHST were made on the third day of administration. The discrepancy between their observations and those in our studies might, therefore, be due to two factors: (1) With the evidence that the pituitary-adrenal mechanism requires longer than three days to adjust to the administration of small doses, some degree of summation effect might be expected on the third day. (2) Because a single oral dose of 12.5 mg of cortisone acetate causes a transient rise in plasma 17-OHST,[25] this might result in a greater increase in urinary steroid excretion than the same amount administered in divided doses.

These investigators also reported that patients receiving 12.5 mg of cortisone acetate twice daily had normal basal plasma 17-OHST levels, indicating that such doses did not produce a

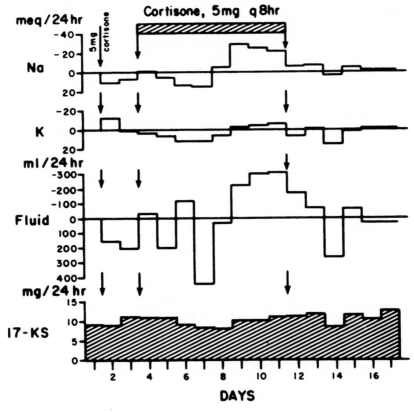

Figure 2. Effects of administration of a single dose of 5 mg of cortisone acetate and of 5 mg every 8 hours for 8 days upon urinary sodium, potassium, fluid, and total neutral 17-ketosteroid (17-KS) excretion. From William McK Jefferies, Low Dosage Glucocorticoid Therapy, *Archives of Internal Medicine, 119*:265-278. Copyright 1967, the American Medical Association. Reprinted by permission.

persistent elevation of plasma cortisol. Nelson and co-workers[25] reported that a single oral dose of 12.5 mg of hydrocortisone caused a peak rise in plasma 17-OHST in one hour with a return to the baseline level by the fourth hour, but the effects of persistent administration of this dosage were not studied. Barbato and Landau[26] demonstrated that 25 mg cortisone acetate or hydrocortisone taken orally produced a peak value of serum cortisol in one to three hours, and by the fifth hour at least one subject had low serum cortisol. A single daily dose of 20 mg of cortisone acetate or hydrocortisone might, therefore, have a different effect on the hypothalamic-pituitary mechanism from the same total amount administered in divided doses throughout the twenty-four-hour period. For this reason, the administration of a single dose of 0.5 mg of dexamethasone[27] or 5 mg of prednisolone[28] in the evening, even though apparently effective in inhibiting adrenocorticotropic hormone and in producing anti-inflammatory effects, may be less physiologic and, therefore, less safe than the low dosage cortisone or hydrocortisone schedule used in our studies. These doses of dexamethasone and prednisolone, being equivalent to approximately 15 mg and 20 mg of hydrocortisone, respectively, represent individual doses three or four times as great as the 5 mg used in our clinic. Their action is probably more similar to that of larger doses administered every other day[29] wherein an intermittent excess of steroid is achieved. Furthermore, the duration of effects of a single dose of the steroid derivatives appears to be longer than that of hydrocortisone, so observations made with natural steroids may not be applicable to derivatives.

It is evident from the above that either replacement or supra-replacement dosages may be hazardous if given for a sufficient period of time, but subreplacement dosages on a divided schedule do not possess such harmful potential.

Why should most physicians be unaware of the safety of the small physiologic dosages? Three major reasons for this are as follows: (1) There has been no promotion of physiologic dosages by pharmaceutical companies. Patents on cortisone and hydrocortisone have expired, and drug regulations require that when a new use is found for an old drug, even at a lower dosage, it must be treated as if it were a new drug and meet all of the investigational requirements of a new drug before the use can be included in the package insert or advertised. Although this requirement is obviously desirable, there is little incentive for a pharmaceutical company to invest the sums necessary to meet these requirements when any competitor could market the drug, especially in the case of medications such as cortisone and hydrocortisone, where such great apprehension exists that a major educational program would be necessary to have the product accepted. (2) There has been little if any discrimination between the effects of physiologic versus pharmacologic dosages. Package inserts for hydrocortisone and cortisone acetate, for example, do not differentiate between physiologic and pharmacologic dosages and effects, implying that any dosage may cause any of the numerous grim side effects that are included in the sections on warnings, precautions, and adverse reactions! This not only causes physicians to be unaware of the safety and proper usage of physiologic dosages but, with the recent emphasis upon package inserts being made available to patients, has caused patients with conditions that require physiologic dosages so as to be able to live normal lives, such as adrenal insufficiency or congenital adrenal hyperplasia, to become so frightened that much reassurance is necessary to convince them that this lifesaving medication is not going to poison them! Thorn described this problem as long ago as 1966,[30] and subsequently it has, if anything, become worse. (3) There is a tendency to confuse cortisone and hydrocortisone with their more potent derivatives, such as prednisone, prednisolone, methyl prednisolone, triamcinolone, and dexamethasone. As noted above, with the profusion of glucocorticoid agents there has been a tendency to term all glucocorticoid therapy "cortisone therapy" regardless of the steroid used. A dosage of 5 mg four times daily of cortisone acetate or hydrocortisone is a safe, physiologic dosage, but 5 mg four times daily of prednisone or any of the other derivatives is at least four times as potent and, hence, subject to all of the hazards of pharmacologic dosages. These and other factors that have contributed to the confusion regarding the safety of glucocorticoid therapy have been reviewed elsewhere.[31]

In addition, some physicians have been discouraged from using smaller dosages of cortisone and hydrocortisone by a report[32] in which it was concluded that "there is no truly physiologic quantity of cortisone, that is, there is no dose of cortisone which on long-term administration to adrenal-deficient patients with or without a small supplement of desoxycorticosterone will not be accompanied by certain signs of hypoadrenalism or certain manifestations of hypercortisonism or both." This conclusion was based on observations of hypertensives who had been subjected to total or subtotal adrenalectomy and who were maintained on minimal dosages of cortisone acetate by mouth. The evidences of adrenal insufficiency were (1) unresponsive hypoglycemia developing at the third and fourth hour of a four-hour glucose tolerance test and (2) abnormal water excretion tests. Such abnormalities need not imply a deficiency in cortisone effectiveness but merely that the minimum maintenance dosage was insufficient to cope with the increased stress of the tests.

The signs of hypercortisonism were "polyphagia, weight gain, and impairment of glucose tolerance." Improvement in appetite is a characteristic effect of cortisone treatment in patients with adrenal insufficiency; this does not necessarily result in excessive weight gain but rather a restoration of normal weight. If excessive weight is gained, the schedule of administration of the steroid may not be optimum, e.g. two doses of 20 mg daily may stimulate the appetite more than four doses of 10 mg, or the subjects may be obesity prone, i.e. possess those unknown metabolic factors that tend to produce obesity in patients without adrenal insufficiency. Impairment of glucose tolerance was noted in only four of seventeen patients tested. This may have resulted from the timing of cortisone administration with relation to the tests in that a dose of 12.5 mg was given just prior to the test; this dosage has been found to be sufficient to cause a transient increase in plasma 17-hydroxycorticosteroids in normal persons,[25] an effect that might produce transient hypercortisonism.

The authors were also concerned that at the end of five years two of the 110 patients adrenalectomized for hypertension had developed frank diabetes mellitus. Subsequent experience has shown that cortisone, even in large doses, does not produce diabetes but merely unmasks it, and it seems likely that the incidence in this series was due to some other factor than the steroid replacement therapy, possibly related to all of these subjects being hypertensives. Because of these points, and also that the doubts regarding the safety of replacement dosages of cortisone have not been substantiated by subsequent clinical experience, at least with divided doses of 10 mg or less, discouragement on the basis of this report is no longer justified.

Perhaps another factor that has contributed to the failure to recognize the value and safety of low dosage glucocorticoid therapy is the inconvenience of having patients take three or four doses daily for optimum effects. This requires more time in the physician's office for explanation of the schedule and more difficulty on the part of patients in following it. Most patients are willing to accept this inconvenience if the reason is explained, especially after they have had an opportunity to experience its beneficial effect. Verbal instructions are often forgotten, so we routinely give printed instructions, an example of which is reproduced, to every patient starting on glucocorticoid therapy. This is reinforced by a discussion in which the patient is encouraged to ask questions. Understanding and cooperation of the patient are essential for this type of therapy and cannot be overemphasized.

The alternate day program for glucocorticoid therapy recommended by Harter, Reddy, and Thorn[29] should be mentioned here to avoid confusion. This schedule was suggested as a method to lessen the occurrence of side effects with large pharmacologic dosages of glucocorticoids. Its chief advantage is a diminution of likelihood of persistent adrenal suppression. Because subreplacement dosages do not produce side effects or complete adrenal suppression, and because they require divided daily doses for optimum effects, there is no reason to administer them on an alternate day schedule.

The investigation of low dosage glucocorticoid therapy has also been handicapped by an attitude on the part of some authorities that everything is known about the clinical effects of cortisone and hydrocortisone, so there is no reason to spend more time and effort studying them further. Such an attitude is not valid because, although much is known about the harmful effects of large doses of glucocorticoids, virtually nothing is known about the mechanism of any of their beneficial clinical actions.

Finally, the possibility of undesirable effects of long-term administration of low doses must be considered. There are several reasons why this is unlikely. First, the uses for which they are given are directed towards restoring normal function rather

INSTRUCTIONS

The medication you have been prescribed is a normal adrenal hormone. In the dosage that you will be taking, it will not cause an excess of hormone in your body or any of the side effects that result from such an excess. You will notice that the tablets taste somewhat bitter; like aspirin, if they are taken on an empty stomach they may cause gastric discomfort and indigestion. It may be helpful, therefore, to take them with milk or with an antacid. If you have ever had a peptic ulcer (of the stomach or duodenum) you should always take an antacid with each dose.

This medication is more effective if you spread out the day's dosage, so you should take_____tablet with each meal and at bedtime, totalling _____ tablets daily. It may be taken before, during, or after meals, but most patients prefer to take it just before meals. If meals are delayed or missed, try to take the medication at the usual mealtime. If you forget to take a dose, for example, at lunchtime, and think of it in the middle of the afternoon, take it when you think of it. If you do not remember it until the next dose is due, take both doses at the same time in order to have the correct total dosage for the day. It will not be harmful to double up on doses, but the medication will be more effective if you take each dose at its proper time. It is helpful to have a small pillbox in which each day's dosage is placed each morning and which is carried with you in your pocket or your handbag, at all times. This not only helps to remind you to take the medication but also will enable you to determine whether you have taken a dose. Sometimes, it is difficult to remember whether you have taken a dose.

Because this is a normal hormone, it will not interfere with your taking any other medication. If you should develop a cold or influenza, double each dose and phone me. You should also take any other medication prescribed by your family physician or by me, such as aspirin, antihistaminics, decongestants, antibiotics, or cough medicine. The increased dosage of this medication should be continued until you have recovered from the infection, then return to your previous dosage.

If any other questions arise, phone my office and ask for my nurse or for me.

William McK. Jefferies, M. D.
Euclid Clinic Foundation
18599 Lake Shore Blvd.
Euclid, Ohio 44119

than altering normal function. Second, the dosages do not produce any excessive steroid level in the blood. Third, although such dosages may affect diurnal variation in plasma cortisol levels, they do not destroy this normal diurnal variation (Fig. 3). Fourth, patients who have been taking subreplacement dosages for long periods respond to ACTH and metyropone comparably to normal subjects.[21] Fifth, there is no evidence that patients who have taken physiologic dosages for as long as twenty-seven years have experienced any harmful effects, nor that children born to women taking physiologic dosages have any increased incidence of congenital defects or other difficulties.

The result of this combination of factors is a unique situation in which a safe therapeutic regimen with promising potential in several broad clinical areas has been practically ignored. A review of the known therapeutic effects of physiologic dosages plus suggestive evidence for even greater therapeutic value in other conditions should at least be convincing of the advisability of further studies.

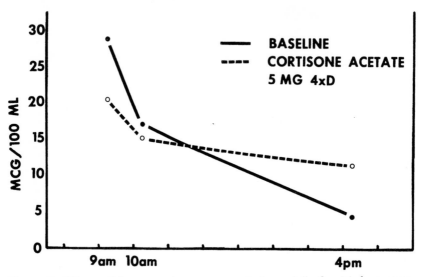

Figure 3. Effects of 5 mg cortisone acetate 4 times daily for 14 days upon diurnal variation of serum 17-hydroxy-corticosteroid levels in a normal male.

REFERENCES

1. Ingle DJ, Baker BL: *Physiological and Therapeutic Effects of Corticotropin (ACTH) and Cortisone.* Springfield, Thomas, 1953, p. 40.
2. Conn JW, Fajans SS, Louis LH, Johnson B: Metabolic and clinical effects of corticosterone (Compound B) in man. In Mote JR (Ed.): *Proceedings of the Second Clinical ACTH Conference.* Vol. I — Research. Philadelphia, Blakiston, 1951, pp. 221-234.
3. Leith W, Beck JC: 9-alpha-fluorohydrocortisone alone and combined with hydrocortisone in the management of chronic adrenal insufficiency. *J Clin Endocrinol Metab 17:*280-290, 1957.
4. Tomas FM, Munro HN, Young VR: Effect of glucocorticoid administration on the rate of muscle protein breakdown in vivo in rats, as measured by urinary excretion of N-methyl-histidine, *Biochem J 178:*139-146, 1979.
5. Perera GA, Pines KL, Hamilton HB, Vislocky K: Clinical and metabolic study of 11-dehydro-17-hydroxycorticosterone acetate (Kendall Compound E) in hypertension, Addison's disease and diabetes mellitus. *Am J Med 7:*56-69, 1949.
6. Thorn GW, Forsham PH: Metabolic changes in man following adrenal and pituitary hormone administration. In Pincus G (Ed.): *Recent Progress in Hormone Research, Vol. IV.* New York, Acad Pr, 1949, pp. 229-288.
7. Thorn GW, Forsham PH, Bennett LL, Roche M, Reiss RS, Slessor A, Flink EB, Somerville W: Clinical and metabolic changes in Addison's disease following administration of Compound E acetate (11-dehydro-17-hydroxycorticosterone acetate). *Trans Assoc Am Physicians 62:*233-244, 1949.
8. Sprague RG, Power MH, Mason HL, Albert A, Mathieson DR, Hench PS, Kendall EC, Slocumb CH, Polley HF: Observations on the physiologic effects of cortisone and ACTH in man. *Arch Intern Med 85:*199-258, 1950.
9. Hench PS, Kendall EC, Slocumb CH, Polley HF: Effects of cortisone acetate and pituitary ACTH on rheumatoid arthritis, rheumatic fever, and certain other conditions. *Arch Intern Med 85:*545-666, 1950.
10. Fourman P, Bartter FC, Albright F, Dempsey EL, Carroll E, Alexander J: Effects of 17-hydroxy-corticosterone (Compound F) in man. *J Clin Invest 29:*1462-1473, 1950.
11. Perera GA, Fleming TC, Pines KL, Crymble M: Cortisone in hypertensive vascular disease. *J Clin Invest 29:*739-744, 1950.
12. Thorn GW, Merrill JP, Smith S III, Roche M, Frawley TF: Clinical studies with ACTH and cortisone in renal disease. *Arch Intern Med 86:*319-354, 1950.
13. Dustan HP, Corcoran AC, Taylor RD, Page IH: Cortisone and ACTH in essential hypertension, establishment of renal glycosuria. *Arch Intern Med 87:*627-635, 1951.

14. Levitt MF, Bader ME: Effect of cortisone and ACTH on fluid and electrolyte distribution in man. *Am J Med 11:*715-723, 1951.

15. Pearson OH, Eliel LP: Experimental studies with ACTH and cortisone in patients with neoplastic disease. In Pincus G, (Ed.): *Recent Progress in Hormone Research, Vol. VI.* New York, Acad Pr, 1951, pp 373-416.

16. Perera GA, Ragan C, Werner SC: Clinical and metabolic study of 17-hydroxycorticosterone (Kendall Compound F); Comparison with cortisone. *Proc Soc Exp Biol Med 77:*326-330, 1951.

17. Sprague RG: Effects of cortisone and ACTH. In Harris, RS, Thimann KV (Eds.); *Vitamins and Hormones, Vol. IX,* New York, Acad Pr, 1951, pp. 265-311.

18. Thorn GW, Renold AE, Wilson DL, Frawley TF, Jenkins D, Garcia-Reyes J, Forsham PH: Clinical studies on activity of orally administered cortisone. *N Engl J Med 245:*549-555, 1951.

19. Sprague RG, Mason HL, Power MH: Physiologic effects of cortisone and ACTH in man. In Pincus G, (Ed.). *Recent Progress in Hormone Research, Vol. VI.* New York, Acad Pr, 1951, pp. 315-365.

20. Garrod O, Burston RA: The diuretic response to ingested water in Addison's disease and panhypopituitarism and the effect of cortisone thereon. *Clin Sci 11:*113-139, 1952.

21. Jefferies WMcK: Low dosage glucocorticoid therapy. *Arch Intern Med 119:*265-278, 1967.

22. Barker MW: The pathologic anatomy in 28 cases of Addison's disease. *Arch Pathol 8:*432-450, 1929.

23. Jefferies WMcK, Kelly LW, Jr., Sydnor KL, Levy RP, Cooper G.: Metabolic effects of a single intravenous infusion of hydrocortisone related to plasma levels in a normal versus an adrenally insufficient subject. *J Clin Endocrinol Metab 17:*186-200, 1957.

24. Shuster S, Williams IA: Pituitary and adrenal function during administration of small doses of corticosteroids. *Lancet 2:*674-678, 1961.

25. Nelson DH, Sandberg AA, Palmer JG, Tyler FH: Blood levels of 17-hydroxy-corticosteroids following administration of adrenal steroids and their relation to levels of circulating leukocytes. *J Clin Invest 31:*843-849, 1952.

26. Barbato AL, Landau RL: Serum cortisol appearance-disappearance in adrenal insufficiency after cortisone acetate. *Acta Endocrinol 84:*600-604, 1977.

27. Nichols T, Nugent CA, Tyler FH: Diurnal variation in suppression of adrenal function by glucocorticoids. *J Clin Endocrinol Metab 25:*343-349, 1965.

28. DeAnrade JR: Pituitary-adrenocortical reserve during corticosteroid therapy: A report on the methopyrapone test in ten patients taking long-continued small doses. *J Clin Endocrinol Metab 24:*261-262, 1964.

29. Harter JG, Reddy WJ, Thorn GW: Studies on an intermittent corticosteroid dosage regimen. *N Engl J Med 269:*591-596, 1963.

30. Thorn GW: Clinical considerations in the use of corticosteroids. *N Engl J Med 274:*775-781, 1966.

31. Jefferies WMcK: Glucocorticoid therapy: An overmaligned reputation with untapped potential benefit. In Inglefinger FJ, Ebert RV, Finland M, Relman AS (Eds.): *Controversies in Internal Medicine II.* Philadelphia, Saunders, 1974, pp. 439-445.

32. Hills AG, Zintel HA, Parsons DW: Observations of human adrenal cortical deficiency. *Am J Med 21:*358-379, 1956.

Chapter 3

THE SIGNIFICANCE OF NORMAL ADRENOCORTICAL FUNCTION

THE ADRENALS are fascinating glands. Situated at the upper pole of each kidney, their significance has been realized only since the 1930s. Early experiments demonstrated that the removal of the adrenals of a rat produced no obvious effect so long as the animal was kept under ideal environmental conditions, viz., proper temperature, proper amounts of food, salt, water and rest at proper intervals, and avoidance of excessive exercise or infection. If any one of these environmental factors was changed, however, the animal died. It therefore became evident that the adrenal glands were necessary for adapting to changes from an ideal environment, that is, to stresses and strains.

Both morphologically and functionally, each adrenal gland consists of two sections; the cortex, or outer portion, and the medulla, or central portion. The hormones of the medulla, epinephrine and norepinephrine, are catecholamines and are primarily involved in acute responses to stress, such as fright, fear, and anger. They are responsible for the increased heart rate, increased blood pressure, and mobilization of sugar from the liver to the blood stream, which prepares the organism for fight or flight.

The hormones of the cortex are steroids of which there are at least four types, and they are essential for the organism's ability to respond to more prolonged stresses such as infection, injury, starvation, and strenuous or prolonged exertion. The most important type of steroid produced by the adrenal cortex is glucocorticoid. This type of steroid has as one of its chief actions stimulation of the conversion of protein to glucose, a process known as gluconeogenesis. This is a vital effect in the maintenance of normal levels of blood glucose when food intake is irregular, since low blood sugar is incompatible with normal

28

function of the brain, muscles, or other tissues of the body. The major glucocorticoid produced in humans is hydrocortisone (cortisol), but cortisone is also produced in small amounts. Cortisone is converted to hydrocortisone before it produces its normal metabolic effects. Glucocorticoids have another action that is of importance in survival under stress, the maintenance of normal vascular tone. The exact mechanisms by which hydrocortisone brings about these critical effects are unknown. For many years hydrocortisone levels in the blood or urine were measured as 17-hydroxycorticosteroids by the Porter-Silber reaction of the 17, 21-dihydroxy, 20-ketones, but radioimmunoassay (RIA) has now made possible more accurate and specific measurements of single steroids.

The second type of adrenocortical hormone is mineralocorticoid, the chief of which is aldosterone. This steroid regulates the levels of sodium and potassium in extra- and intracellular fluid, respectively, promoting sodium retention and potassium loss, an action that is necessary for normal fluid and electrolyte balance and for maintenance of normal blood pressure. Natural glucocorticoids also have some electrolyte-regulating effect.

The third type is androgen, represented by dehydroepiandrosterone and androstenedione, and their chief function appears to be promotion of growth and repair of protein tissues of the body, especially muscle. This effect is important not only in normal growth and development but also in healing of tissue damaged by injury or infection. Until recently, androgen levels were estimated by urinary excretion of 17-ketosteroids (17-KS), a relatively nonspecific method, since not all androgens are excreted as 17-KS and not all 17-KS are metabolites of androgens. As with glucocorticoids, radioimmunoassay is now replacing earlier methods.

The fourth type is estrogen. Adrenal estrogen seems to be mainly involved in providing a supply of this hormone during menses and at the menopause when production by the ovaries is temporarily or permanently interrupted, but it may have other, as yet unrecognized functions in growth or development. Some estrogen is produced directly in the adrenals, but estrogen may also be produced in peripheral tissues from dehydroepiandrosterone, one of the androgens produced in the adrenal cortex.

A fifth type of hormone produced by the adrenal cortex seems quite likely, but the evidence for its existence is only indirect, and its chemical identity is not known. This possible hormone has an anti-sodium-retaining, or natriuretic, effect. It has been recognized for many years that patients with adrenal insufficiency not only are more susceptible to low levels of serum sodium, with resulting hypotension and shock, but are also more susceptible to pathologic sodium retention from excessive amounts of salt or of sodium-retaining steroids such as aldosterone, desoxycorticosterone, or 9-alpha-fluorohydrocortisone, suggesting that the adrenals may produce a substance that protects against excessive sodium retention.

In 1948 Wilkins and Lewis[1] suggested that a steroid promoting sodium excretion might exist, as an explanation for the excessive salt loss that occurs in some patients with congenital adrenal hyperplasia. Experimental evidence for this possibility was reported in 1949 by Knowlton and his associates.[2] After producing cytotoxic serum nephritis in rats, they found that injections of 2.5 mg cortisone acetate daily in nonadrenalectomized animals produced a moderate hypertension, whereas injections into adrenalectomized animals caused severe hypertension. Jailer[3] summarized evidence for this salt-losing adrenal hormone in 1951, and Cope[4] provided a more recent summary in 1972.

Two hormones produced normally by ovaries, progesterone and 17-hydroxyprogesterone, have been demonstrated to have natriuretic properties,[5-8] and they are known intermediary steroids in adrenal cortices in the pathway of production of hydrocortisone, occurring in excess in certain types of congenital adrenal hyperplasia, but the possibility that they may aid in normal water balance has not apparently been investigated.

The identification of normal anti-sodium-retaining factors would be of special interest because of their possible relation to some cases of hypertension. In addition to hypertension being caused by excessive sodium-retaining hormones such as aldosterone and desoxycorticosterone, it might also result from a deficiency of sodium-excreting factors.

In the unstressed state a diurnal pattern of production of gluco-corticoid and androgen occurs. A person who sleeps from 11 PM to 7 AM has a maximum level of hydrocortisone in his blood at approximately 8 AM, then it gradually decreases through the day and evening, reaching a low point at approximately 1 AM, following which it increases progressively during sleep to reach its maximum again at 8 AM the next day. The peak level of plasma cortisol in a normal individual is usually between 20 and 30 mcg/100 ml, and the lowest level is approximately 5 to 10 mcg/100 ml. This diurnal pattern is related to a person's sleep-wake schedule, and when this schedule is changed, as occurs when a person changes from one work shift to another, or when one travels to different time zones, approximately five to ten days are required before a stable new diurnal pattern of plasma cortisol level is reached. This is apparently a major factor responsible for travel fatigue or "jet lag" and suggests that industries that change the time schedules of their workers frequently may not be achieving maximum work effort from them but may actually be impairing their efficiency. A recent survey found that workers on rotating shifts suffered a significantly higher incidence of illness and became more accident-prone.

The significance of the diurnal pattern of cortico-steroid production is not definitely known, but it is apparently related to nature's plan for restoring energy by a period of sleep in each twenty-four hours. It seems that we need a period of about eight hours sleep in each twenty-four hours to recharge our batteries. The circadian periodicity of corticosteroid production occurs in animals also. There is evidence that in the rat this periodicity becomes established twenty-one to twenty-five days after birth, but it may be suppressed by administration of corticosteroids between days two and four of neonatal life,[9] suggesting that administration of excessive dosages of glucocorticoids to infants may permanently affect their pituitary or adrenocortical function.

STRESS

The importance of the adrenal cortex in response to stress is indicated by studies of the general adaptation syndrome. This is the sum of the organism's nonspecific response to stress and has been intensively studied and described by Selye.[10] It consists of three main stages: the alarm reaction, the stage of resistance, and the stage of exhaustion. The third stage comes into play only if the alarming stimulus is sufficiently severe and sufficiently prolonged.

The alarm reaction has been divided into an initial stage of shock and a secondary stage of countershock. Evidence indicates that during the initial stage of shock, effects characteristic of an acute release of epinephrine are followed by changes characteristic of relative adrenocortical insufficiency (a fall in blood pressure, decreased blood sugar, decreased blood sodium, and increased blood potassium) lasting a few minutes to hours. The stage of countershock then occurs, with effects characteristic of increased adrenocorticoid activity (return of blood pressure to normal or above normal; increased blood sugar; restoration of normal or increased level of blood sodium and normal or decreased level of blood potassium; and enlargement of the adrenal cortex). These effects return to baseline during the stage of resistance but reappear during the stage of exhaustion. In hypophysectomized animals these changes do not occur, indicating that they are mediated by the hypothalamus and pituitary gland through their production of corticotropin releasing factor (CRF) and adrenocorticotrophic hormone (ACTH), respectively. During the recovery phase, and as the production of hydrocortisone returns to normal, the production of androgens increases and apparently is related to the healing process. It is therefore evident that adrenocortical hormones, especially hydrocortisone, play an important role in normal response to stress.

The critical role of the adrenal cortex in response to stress in human subjects is manifested in a number of ways. A patient with untreated mild adrenal insufficiency or low adrenal reserve may function reasonably well when environmental conditions are optimum but tends to tire more easily, and if strenuous physical exercise is undertaken or a meal skipped, hypoglycemic symptoms or convulsions may develop. If an infection such as a common cold develops, acute adrenal insufficiency with nausea, vomiting, a falling blood pressure, and collapse may occur. All of these undesirable developments may be prevented by administration of suitable dosages of hydrocortisone. It has also been demonstrated that normal adrenocortical function is essential for ability to withstand infections, several studies having indicated that either too little or too much glucocorticoid can impair resistance to infection, whereas an optimum level of glucocorticoid enhances resistance to infection.[11, 12]

In addition to the importance of the adrenals in response to stress as a factor in survival, the effects of the adrenocortical steroids upon growth and maturation may account for many of the differences in physical development and energy between individuals. It has been found, for example, that each person has his or her own characteristic pattern of urinary 17-ketosteroid fractions,[13] and it appears likely that this pattern is related to physical development.

From the time that steroid fractions were first measured in pooled urine from individual subjects, a constancy of pattern for each person has been noted.[14, 15] In 1963 Michelakis and I[13] confirmed, through a different fractionation technique on twenty-four-hour urine collections, that normal individuals have reproducible patterns of excretion of 17-KS fractions. In addition we found that women with hirsutism or ovarian dysfunction had reproducible individual patterns. It therefore appears that each person tends to have a characteristic level of excretion of each 17-KS fraction and a reproducible pattern of excretions of these fractions in the unstressed state, but significant variations of pattern occur between normal persons as well as between patients.

After administration of small doses of ACTH or corticosteroid it became evident that some persons may have variations in pattern with different degrees of ACTH stimulation.[13] Although some subjects respond to a standard ACTH stimulus with a uniform rise in all fractions, in others the responses are asymmetrical, with variations in rise of excretions of different fractions from an insignificant amount to an increment far greater than average. Such differences could result from differences in production by the adrenals of steroids that are metabolized and excreted as 17-KS in the urine, or from differences in metabolism of 17-KS precursors in the liver or other tissues.

It is therefore evident that in some persons fluctuations in endogenous ACTH may alter steroid excretion patterns, whereas in others they may not. Hirsutism and acne are known to result from excess androgen, and excess estrogen can cause ovarian dysfunction. Although there is evidence that the occurrence of hirsutism, acne, or ovarian dysfunction is not necessarily related to any single specific pattern of steroid excretion,[13] the variation of pattern with different levels of ACTH stimulation may be related to the clinical observation that women may develop hirsutism, acne, or ovarian dysfunction after stress.

In 1964, Prezio et al.[16] reported that resting urinary 17-hydroxycorticosteroid (17-OHST) levels correlated with lean body mass, whereas after ACTH stimulation the best correlation of 17-OHST excretion was with excess fat and total body weight, suggesting that adrenal production of glucocorticoids was related to body size and fat composition. Dunkelman and his associates[17] found that obese persons not only had increased urinary 17-OHST compared with nonobese controls but cortisol production rates were also high, plasma cortisol levels tended to be high, and response to a standard ACTH stimulus was greater than normal.

These studies suggest that individual differences in steroid production or metabolism may significantly influence body growth and development, and it is quite likely that they may affect the aging process, response to stress, and possibly even the development of "stress diseases." The adrenals undoubtedly contribute significantly to the factors that make us different individuals.

REFERENCES

1. Wilkins L, Lewis RA: The renal excretion of steroid hormones in pseudohermaphroditism and male sexual precocity associated with symptoms of Addison's disease. In Reifenstein EC, Jr., (Ed.): *Trans 17th Conf Metabolic Aspects of Convalescence.* New York, Josiah Macy, Jr. Fndn, 1948, pp. 168-174.
2. Knowlton AI, Loeb EM, Stoerk HC, Seegal BC: The development of hypertension and nephritis in normal and adrenalectomized rats treated with cortisone. *Proc Soc Exp Biol Med* 72:722-725, 1949.

3. Jailer JW: Evidence for a "salt-losing" adrenal hormone in congenital adrenal virilism associated with Addisonian-like symptoms. *J Clin Endocrinol 11:*798, 1951.

4. Cope CL: *Adrenal Steroids and Disease,* 2nd ed., Philadelphia, Lippincott, 1972, pp. 434-438.

5. Landau RL, Lugibihl K: Inhibition of the sodium-retaining influence of aldosterone by progesterone. *J Clin Endocrinol Metab 18:*1237-1245, 1958.

6. Jacobs DR, Van Der Poll J, Gabrilove JL, Soffer LJ: 17α-Hydroxy-progesterone — a salt-losing steroid: Relation to congenital adrenal hyperplasia. *J Clin Endocrinol Metab 21:*909-922, 1961.

7. Laidlaw JC, Ruse JL, Gornall AG: The influence of estrogen and progesterone on aldosterone excretion. *J Clin Endocrinol Metab 22:*161-171, 1962.

8. Jacobs DR: Natriuretic activity of 17-hydroxyprogesterone in man. *Acta Endocrinol 61:*275-282, 1969.

9. Krieger DT: Circadian corticosteroid periodicity: critical period for abolition by neonatal injection of corticosteroid. *Science 178:*1205-1207, 1972.

10. Selye H: The general adaptation syndrome and diseases of adaptation. *J Clin Endocrinol Metab 6:*117-230, 1946.

11. Kass EH, Finland M: Corticosteroids and infections. *Adv Intern Med 9:*45-80, 1958.

12. Beisel WR, Rapoport MI: Interrelations between adrenocortical functions and infectious illness. *N Engl J Med 280:*541-546, 596-604, 1969.

13. Jefferies WMcK, Michelakis AM: Individual patterns of urinary 17-ketosteroid fractions. *Metabolism 12:*1017-1031, 1963.

14. Dobriner K: Studies in steroid metabolism, XX. The reproductibility of urinary steroid patterns in humans. *J Clin Invest 32:*950-951, 1953.

15. Kappas A, Gallagher TF: Studies in steroid metabolism XXVIII. The alpha-ketosteroid excretion pattern in normal females and the response to ACTH. *J Clin Invest 34:*1566-1572, 1955.

16. Prezio JA, Carreon G, Clerkin E, Meloni CR, Kyle LH, Canary JH: Influence of body composition on adrenal function in obesity. *J Clin Endocrinol Metab 24:*481-485, 1964.

17. Dunkelman SS, Fairhurst B, Plager J, Waterhouse C: Cortisol metabolism in obesity. *J Clin Endocrinol Metab 24:*832-841, 1964.

Chapter 4

ACCEPTED USES OF
PHYSIOLOGIC DOSAGES

ADRENAL INSUFFICIENCY

THE MOST LOGICAL use of physiologic dosages of cortisone or hydrocortisone is in the treatment of patients with adrenal insufficiency. Severe examples of this disorder are manifested by hyperpigmentation of the skin, weakness, fatigue, anorexia, and susceptibility to collapse and shock with exposure to stress. This clinical picture was first described by Sir Thomas Addison in 1855 and, hence, has been called Addison's disease. For many years tuberculosis of the adrenals was its most frequent cause, but with the decreased incidence of tuberculosis resulting from improved prevention and treatment, "idiopathic" adrenal insufficiency is a more common diagnosis today. In many cases adrenal insufficiency seems to result from a type of autoimmune phenomenon.[1] Improved methods of diagnosis have resulted in the identification of milder degrees of adrenal insufficiency in which the classical clinical picture is incomplete. The mildest form is low adrenal reserve, in which the adrenals are capable of producing sufficient hormone to maintain an apparently normal state of health in the absence of stress, but with increased demand for adrenocortical hormone, symptoms, or even collapse, may occur.

Because chronic fatigue is frequently the earliest symptom of mild adrenal insufficiency and with the availability of a simple and reliable method of determining adrenal responsiveness to ACTH on an ambulatory basis, patients coming to our clinic complaining of chronic fatigue without other evident cause such as inadequate rest, anemia, hypothyroidism, or chronic illness of any type have been given ACTH tests. These tests have been performed as follows:

Blood is drawn for a baseline plasma cortisol level, recording the time of day. Although it is preferable to perform the test in

36

the morning when plasma cortisol levels are highest if the patient is on a normal sleep-wake schedule, adrenal responsiveness can be determined at any time of the day. The patient does not have to be fasting, but he or she should not have taken any glucocorticoid for at least twelve hours, and preferably not for several weeks, because an abnormal ACTH test due to low adrenal reserve may return to normal after a short course of cortisone acetate or hydrocortisone, and evidence of low reserve may not return until medication has been withdrawn for several weeks. After the blood for baseline plasma cortisol is drawn, the patient receives an injection of 25 units of ACTH of a type that is rapidly absorbed, in contrast to ACTH gel, which is very slowly absorbed. In our clinic we use Cortrosyn®, an active ACTH fraction consisting of twelve amino acids, which has a relatively rapid effect, enabling the test to be run in thirty minutes.[2] If lyophilized ACTH is given, an interval of an hour is preferable to determine adrenal response. After the thirty minutes or one hour interval, depending upon the type of ACTH administered, a second blood specimen is drawn for plasma cortisol determination. A normal response consists of an increase to at least double the baseline value. Most normal persons will have a greater than twofold increase. Although it is possible that patients may have some diminution of adrenal reserve while still demonstrating a twofold response to ACTH, for the present this seems to be a practical point at which to diagnose low adrenal reserve. Others[2, 3, 4] have used different criteria for defining normal adrenal response, but they employed a different method for measuring plasma cortisol levels with a lower normal range. Cortrosyn has a theoretical advantage of being less apt to cause reactions in persons allergic to some ingredient in the injection, but in our experience no significant reactions have been encountered with either Cortrosyn or lyophilized ACTH.

When plasma cortisols are determined by radioimmunoassay, as is done in our laboratory, baseline plasma cortisol values normally lie between 15 and 30 mcg/100 ml in the morning and between 5 and 15 mcg/100 ml in the afternoon.

This test is an example of the impossibility of having strict end points in designating normal ranges of hormone levels, since a normal range can depend upon so many factors. For example, patients with adrenal insufficiency may have plasma cortisol levels within low normal range, especially in the afternoon and evening, and patients with hyperadrenalism may have plasma cortisol levels within normal limits in the morning. It is possible that milder degrees of low adrenal reserve may not be detected unless ACTH tests are performed in the morning at a time when the baseline cortisol levels are maximum.

It is also important to bear in mind that normal ranges for baseline levels of plasma cortisol have been determined by measurements on apparently normal subjects who had no clinical evidence of hyperadrenalism (Cushing's syndrome), hypoadrenalism (Addison's disease), congenital adrenal hyperplasia (adrenogenital syndrome), or other apparent illness. As is evident from subsequent discussion, adrenal dysfunction can be present in many persons who do not fall into any of the above groups, hence so-called "normal" ranges are probably greater than those that would be obtained by excluding, for example, any subject with acne, hirsutism, or allergies, conditions that may have associated mild disorders of adrenocortical function. The normal range used in our laboratory is based on measurements in a relatively small number of subjects who seemed to meet more strict criteria for normalcy, but the number of such subjects encountered in my consulting practice is not sufficiently great for statistical validity. This number obviously should be extended. Meanwhile, the normal range employed is the best that has been available.

Adrenal insufficiency is also characterized by an elevated plasma ACTH level, but patients with low adrenal reserve may have normal plasma ACTH, so the ACTH test of adrenal response is a more sensitive method of diagnosing low adrenal reserve.

Because spontaneous adrenal insufficiency results from progressive destruction of adrenal tissue, symptoms appear when the process reaches the point where remaining adrenal tissue is insufficient to maintain normal well-being. As mentioned previously, this may require destruction of over 90 percent of the glandular tissue, but the remnant is capable of some function, so replacement dosages of cortisone acetate or hydrocortisone in chronic adrenal insufficiency are usually less than the 35-40 mg daily that are required for the totally adrenalectomized patient. Most patients can be maintained on between 20 and 30 mg daily in divided doses. Although some patients may feel well on less than 20 mg daily, it seems preferable to give at least this much hydrocortisone, even to patients with low adrenal reserve, because it takes the strain off of the residual adrenal tissue and provides for more functional reserve in times of stress. Under some circumstances, it appears to provide an opportunity for residual tissue to regenerate. A few patients with low reserve have demonstrated evidence of recovery of reserve after months or even years of such treatment, but most seem to require some replacement for the remainder of their lives.

In patients with adrenal insufficiency secondary to tuberculosis, the administration of cortisone or hydrocortisone was initially employed with hesitation because of the well-known anti-inflammatory effect of large doses of glucocorticoids, causing a tendency for tubercles to break down and enable dissemination of the previously walled-off tubercle bacilli. Later, when it was found that the use of glucocorticoids in conjunction with anti-tuberculous therapy actually enhances the effectiveness of the latter, the combined use of the two types of therapy became accepted practice. A patient with adrenal insufficiency secondary to tuberculous infection, therefore, should initially receive a suitable course of antituberculous therapy in addition to replacement cortisone or hydrocortisone.

A schedule of replacement glucocorticoid therapy in adrenal insufficiency employing two-thirds of the daily dosage before breakfast and one-third before supper has been widely recommended.[5] This is based upon the characteristic diurnal variation in plasma cortisol levels, with a peak shortly after waking in the morning and a low point shortly after retiring at night. Patients with adrenal insufficiency will do fairly well on this schedule, but when we have had them compare it with the same total dosage in four divided doses, they have invariably preferred the latter. This is not surprising in view of the evidence that the half-life of hydrocortisone in the blood is only 100 minutes, and some metabolic effects of even large doses do not last longer than eight hours.[6] Furthermore, although plasma cortisol reaches its lowest level shortly after retiring in the evening, it begins to rise during sleep so that by the time the patient arises in the morning it is almost at its peak for the twenty-four-hour period. Hence, instead of the twice daily dosage more closely imitating the natural diurnal pattern, it causes a peak level in the morning followed by a period of lower than normal levels in the afternoon, then a smaller peak after supper followed by a lower than normal level during sleep and at the time of awakening in the morning. The patient is, therefore, relatively adrenally insufficient both in the afternoon and in the early morning. It is not surprising that a schedule employing four doses taken before meals and at bedtime produces more energy and less fatigue.

A four times daily schedule also seems to result in greater decrease in pigmentation. It is therefore possible that a schedule of only two doses daily may not produce sufficient feedback to prevent excessive ACTH production, and this may contribute to the tendency for some patients on this program to develop pituitary adenomas (Nelson's syndrome). Unless and until a longer acting preparation of cortisone or hydrocortisone is made available, a four times daily schedule will, therefore, be preferable to a two times daily schedule. Furthermore, although a lower dosage at supper time is logical and seems to diminish a tendency to insomnia that occurs in some patients, a low dosage at bedtime is not necessarily rational because with normal diurnal variation the plasma cortisol level rises during sleep to reach a peak shortly after awakening in the morning.

An undesirable effect of taking any dosage of glucocorticoid at bedtime is that it tends to cause persistent renal function during sleep, resulting in the need to get up to void once or twice during the night. This is not a serious problem, and most patients prefer this inconvenience to the morning fatigue that may result from an inadequate dose of steroid at bedtime. If the patient has sufficient adrenal reserve, the bedtime dosage may be decreased or omitted entirely without difficulty.

The occasional patient who complains of inability to sleep after the bedtime dosage of glucocorticoid may be found to be taking it without any milk or food, and the insomnia appears to be related to a tendency to acid indigestion aggravated by the steroid. Such a complaint can usually be corrected by taking an antacid or milk or other light nourishment at the time of the bedtime dosage.

Also, insomnia after the bedtime dosage may be related to an excessive intake of coffee or other caffeine-containing beverages that patients with chronic fatigue frequently resort to in an attempt to obtain more energy. Patients with untreated or inadequately treated adrenal insufficiency seem to be tolerant of larger amounts of caffeine; when suitable replacement dosages of cortisone acetate or hydrocortisone are administered, the tolerance returns towards normal, and they may develop symptoms of excessive caffeine intake. It is, therefore, wise to caution patients who are starting on physiologic doses of glucocorticoid regarding this possibility.

Patients with chronic adrenal insufficiency can usually be well maintained with cortisone acetate or hydrocortisone, 5 or 7.5 mg orally before each meal and at bedtime. If a patient has a peptic ulcer or predisposition to this disorder, antacid should be taken with each dose. If this is done, the administration of physiologic dosages of cortisone acetate or hydrocortisone may be continued with suitable ulcer therapy without preventing healing of the ulcer.[7, 8] Several patients with peptic ulcers or tendencies to acid indigestion have stated that cortisone acetate causes less gastric distress than hydrocortisone. Otherwise, there appears to be no significant advantage of either of these steroids over the other. Printed instructions, such as those in Chapter 2, are advisable for patients to keep in a prominent place at home where they can be referred to easily.

Patients who have been totally adrenalectomized can be maintained on cortisone acetate or hydrocortisone in a dosage of 10 mg at breakfast and lunch, 5 mg at supper, and 10 mg at bedtime. Supplementary sodium-retaining activity is usually necessary, and 9-α-fluorohydrocortisone (9-alpha-FF), 0.05 to 0.1 mg daily or every other day, is sufficient in most cases. Patients with spontaneous chronic adrenal insufficiency may not require supplementary sodium-retaining steroid unless they are given one of the derivatives of the natural glucocorticoids that has less sodium-retaining activity. Prednisone, prednisolone, triamcinolone, methyl prednisolone, or dexamethasone are therefore less satisfactory in the treatment of adrenal insufficiency, where all of the physiologic properties of cortisone and hydrocortisone, including sodium retention, are needed.

Rarely, a patient is encountered who is allergic to one of the ingredients used by pharmaceutical companies in the filler for tablets of cortisone acetate or hydrocortisone, developing an allergic dermatitis whenever these tablets are taken in physiologic dosage. Pharmacologic dosages, by contrast, protect against this as well as other allergic manifestations. In such cases, change to a preparation of another pharmaceutical manufacturer may be tolerated. We have encountered one patient who had to be given hydrocortisone liquid, or specially prepared capsules, to avoid such allergic complications.

In addition to supplementary sodium-retaining activity as provided by small doses of 9-alpha-FF, women with adrenal insufficiency often require supplementary androgen to achieve optimum strength and sense of well-being. This is not surprising, since their sole source of androgen is normally the adrenals. Unfortunately, natural adrenal androgens such as dehydroepiandrosterone and androstenedione are not available for clinical use, so small doses of testosterone or one of the other commercially available androgens must be given. Methyl testosterone or fluoxymesterone may be taken orally and, hence, are the most convenient. Five mg daily is usually adequate. As will be discussed later, there is evidence that dehydroepiandrosterone is a better replacement steroid for adrenal insufficiency than testosterone or other androgens.

When a patient with adrenal insufficiency encounters stress, additional cortisone acetate or hydrocortisone is necessary to maintain normal health and sense of well-being. This can vary from the extra 10 mg that may be taken by the businessman who has an unusually strenuous day ahead to the several hundred milligrams per day that may be required in the presence of an acute overwhelming infection. When a patient needs additional steroid, he or she first notices a sensation of fatigue that will disappear as soon as sufficient hydrocortisone is taken. If supplementary glucocorticoid is not taken, the fatigue may progress to malaise and generalized aching similar to that experienced when a person is developing influenza. If additional steroid is still not taken, nausea, vomiting, and collapse with a high fever, fall in blood pressure, and shock may ensue. This condition has been termed "adrenal crisis." Under such circumstances, the amount of cortisone or hydrocortisone necessary to restore a sense of well-being with normal vital signs is physiologic regardless of the dosage. Such a patient will usually respond satisfactorily to 50 mg hydrocortisone sodium succinate (Solu-Cortef®) by intravenous (IV) push, followed by 100 mg in 1000 ml 5 percent dextrose in saline by continuous IV drip over eight hours. This should be followed by additional Solu-Cortef intramuscularly every six hours in doses dependent upon the patient's response. The intramuscular route is preferable except in cases of circulatory collapse in that it permits more flexibility of intravenous therapy, and it is continued until the patient can tolerate oral medication.

Hydrocortisone sodium succinate is more satisfactory for this type of intramuscular replacement therapy than cortisone acetate because cortisone acetate is more slowly absorbed, requiring several hours to reach therapeutic blood levels. If the patient is unable to take oral nourishment, supplementary potassium should be given parenterally after the first liter of IV fluid to prevent hypokalemia. This can be satisfactorily achieved by adding 15 mEq potassium chloride (KCl) to each liter of intravenous fluid after the first until the patient is able to take oral nourishment containing potassium, such as broth or orange juice. The sodium-retaining effect of these dosages of hydrocortisone is sufficient so that supplementary sodium-retaining steroid is not necessary.

After the patient feels well, the dosage of hydrocortisone may usually be rapidly tapered to a maintenance level depending upon the nature of the stress causing the acute insufficiency. If the dosage is not tapered sufficiently promptly, the patient may develop a transient psychosis of a "toxic" type or hypokalemia sufficient to cause weakness. The latter may be mistaken for evidence of an inadequate amount of glucocorticoid, and if more is given, the patient's condition will worsen instead of improve. If there is any question, a serum potassium level should be obtained, or an electrocardiogram, which will show characteristic changes with potassium deficiency, should be run. As soon as the patient feels well, therefore, it is advisable to taper the dose of steroid to a maintenance level as quickly as possible. Often this can be done within twenty-four hours. Hence, a patient with adrenal insufficiency under stress requires dosages of hydrocortisone to maintain a physiologic state that would produce hypercortisonism with its well-known undesirable effects in the unstressed state.

Patients with adrenal insufficiency should, therefore, be told to take extra hydrocortisone when they begin to feel unusually fatigued. If they seem to be developing a respiratory infection, they should be instructed to increase their daily maintenance dosage depending upon the severity of symptoms, and they should take additional steroid until a sense of well-being is restored. If their illness is associated with nausea and vomiting, such as "intestinal flu" or acute gastroenteritis, hydrocortisone must be given parenterally, the sooner the better. For this reason patients with adrenal insufficiency should always have vials of hydrocortisone (with sterile needles and syringes) for parenteral administration in their homes, or if they are traveling, in their personal luggage, and they and members of their families should be instructed in their use.

Because it is difficult to obtain medications away from home, patients should be advised to take at least two supplies of their medications, including hydrocortisone sodium succinate (Solu-Cortef, the Upjohn Company) in Mix-O-Vials®, when they are traveling. One supply should be packed with their luggage, and one should be carried on their person. Hence, if one is lost, the other is available. This is especially important on trips outside the United States. This is another situation in which I have found that printed instructions are helpful.

Patients with adrenal insufficiency should also be cautioned to carry identification cards indicating their diagnosis, treatment, and the name, address, and telephone number of the physician

INSTRUCTIONS FOR PATIENTS TRAVELING

1. Plan to take at least two complete supplies of every medication you are taking. In other words, if you are taking one tablet 4 times daily and are going to be away for two weeks, you will need 14 x 4 = 56 tablets for your trip. Therefore take at least 60 tablets in each of the two containers (total 120 tablets). One should be carried with you in a pocket or in a handbag, and the other should be packed in your luggage. Hence, if one is lost, the other will be available. It is extremely difficult to get a new supply of medication away from home, especially if you are on a trip outside of the United States.

2. If you have adrenal insufficiency or low adrenal reserve, you should take at least 2 Mix-O-Vials of Solu-Cortef with syringes and needles and alcohol for intramuscular injection. If you do not know how to administer intramuscular injection, have my nurse instruct you. Carry one vial with you and pack one in your luggage.

3. If you have diabetes mellitus and are taking insulin, you should take at least two supplies of insulin with syringes, needles, and alcohol, also carried and packed as above.

4. If you have diabetes mellitus or adrenal insufficiency or are allergic to any medications, you should carry some evidence of this at all times, such as a prescription blank indicating your diagnosis and treatment or a Medic-Alert bracelet. Then if you become ill or have an accident away from home, the doctor treating you will have this important information.

to be notified in case of emergency. Medic-Alert (The Medic-Alert Foundation, P.O. Box 1009, Turlock, California 95380) bracelets or necklaces are very good for this type of identification. Such information might be lifesaving in case of an accident in which the patient is rendered unconscious, and it is always helpful for any physician who does not know the patient's background.

When patients with adrenal insufficiency are treated according to these principles, they can live perfectly normal, healthy lives. In some respects they seem to be healthier than many persons without adrenal insufficiency in that they often appear to have more energy, less fatigue, and a greater resistance to at least some types of infection. This will be discussed in greater detail later, but at this point it should be noted that when adrenally insufficient patients with common respiratory infections are treated according to these principles, no increased incidence of complications occurs, and antibiotic therapy is not necessary unless a bacterial infection is present.

A review of several case histories may be helpful in understanding some of the therapeutic points that have been mentioned.

Case 1

The first patient with adrenal insufficiency to be treated with cortisone in our clinic was a young woman who was seen initially in 1949 at the age of twenty-nine years complaining of progressive weakness, malaise, and diarrhea of approximately six months duration. Increased pigmentation of her skin, absence of axillary hair, and low blood pressure strongly suggested adrenal insufficiency, and failure to respond to ACTH with a decrease in circulating eosinophils was consistent with that diagnosis. Present methods of measuring plasma cortisol and ACTH were not available then. There was no history of tuberculosis or evidence of this disease, so a diagnosis of Addison's disease of unknown etiology was made.

The patient was initially treated with desoxycorticosterone acetate pellets implanted subcutaneously, plus increased salt intake and frequent feedings. Later, methyl testosterone, one 5 mg. linguet daily, was added with considerable improvement in her strength and energy. In 1951 when cortisone acetate became available for general clinical use, it was added to her therapy, but because she was our first patient with adrenal insufficiency to receive this medication for maintenance therapy, an optimum dosage schedule was not known.

Initially the patient was told to take a single dose of 12.5 mg daily. Later this was increased to 12.5 mg twice daily with impressive symptomatic improvement, then to 12.5 mg every eight hours with further improvement, but she did not reach an optimum clinical state until she received a dosage of 10 mg before each meal and 5 mg at bedtime. In 1957, 9-alpha-FF was given orally in place of the subcutaneous desoxycorticosterone pellets, and a dosage of 0.05 mg three times weekly achieved adequate supplementary sodium-retaining effect while she was receiving the 35 mg of cortisone acetate.

The patient was told to double her dosage of cortisone acetate in the event of the development of an upper respiratory infection, but later it became evident that an increase in dosage to 80 mg daily (20 mg four times daily) enabled her to recover from respiratory infections more quickly, and an increase to 120 mg (30 mg four times daily) enabled her to withstand an attack of acute influenza without serious problems. The patient's previous history was interesting in that after she had had one full-term delivery her menstrual periods had stopped several years before she developed symptoms of adrenal insufficiency.

Urinary gonadotropin excretion was normal. A dosage of 1.25 mg of conjugated estrogens daily for three weeks on and one week off produced regular withdrawal menstrual flow. At age forty-five, urinary gonadotropins were elevated, so cyclic Premarin®,* 1.25 mg daily, was continued until age fifty-six. She is now fifty-eight years old and apparently healthy with normal energy and strength.

This patient demonstrated the benefit of androgen administration to women with adrenal insufficiency, with further improvement from cortisone acetate, but this had to be given in four divided doses to achieve an optimum therapeutic effect. Her clinical course also demonstrated that an increase in cortisone dosage to 80 mg daily enabled her to recover from respiratory infections with little difficulty, and an increase to 120 mg daily enabled her to withstand acute influenza without serious problems. With the now known relationship between adrenocortical and ovarian function, it is possible that her amenorrhea may have been related to her adrenal disorder, but replacement dosages of estrogen were continued up to the menopause, so there was no opportunity to observe whether normal ovarian function might have resumed with cortisone therapy in a manner similar to that of other patients (Cases 3 and 4). She further demonstrates that a patient with adrenal insufficiency can live a relatively normal life with suitable replacement therapy, since she is still quite well twenty-nine years after the condition was diagnosed.

Case 2

This case is an example of a combination of several hormone disorders, including primary adrenal insufficiency. The patient is a fifty-seven year old woman who at age seventeen had a hyperactive goiter removed surgically. About two years later she developed malaise and easy fatigue and began having upper respiratory infections that lasted a month or more. At age twenty-two she developed acute appendicitis; when an appendectomy was performed, she suffered postoperative collapse, but she recovered with general supportive measures.

Easy fatigue and frequent respiratory infections persisted, until at age twenty-seven a diagnosis of Addison's disease was made. No prior history of tuberculosis in the patient or in her family was known. Desoxycorticosterone acetate pellets were implanted subcutaneously. Menses were somewhat irregular. She was married at age twenty-nine,

---

* A list of generic names for proprietary pharmaceuticals mentioned in the text appears in the Appendix, pp. 181-183.

used no precautions, but had no pregnancies. In 1953, at age thirty-two, cortisone acetate therapy was started at another clinic in a dosage of 12.5 mg every twelve hours with occasional increase for malaise. She not only felt better but had no respiratory infections for the next six or seven years. At age forty a recurrence of hyperthyroidism was treated with radioactive iodine.

At age forty-seven, shortly after she was referred to me, she had an attack of influenza with a temperature of 102°. Her cortisone dosage was increased to 12.5 mg four times daily, and she recovered uneventfully. She felt so much better during her convalescence when she was taking 7.5 mg of hydrocortisone four times daily that this dosage was continued. She not only had more energy than she had while taking 12.5 mg twice daily, but her skin pigmentation decreased for the first time. Because hypothyroidism developed following radioactive iodine treatment, l-thyroxine (Synthroid®), 0.05 mg daily, was added.

At age forty-nine a nodule was noted in the right breast, and at surgery, which was undertaken less than a week after the nodule was first noted, carcinoma was found in both breasts with metastatic involvement of the nodes in the left axilla. A bilateral radical mastectomy was performed, followed by postoperative radiation therapy to the axillae and chest. At the time of surgery, supplementary hydrocortisone sodium succinate was administered in a dosage of 100 mg intramuscularly one hour preoperatively and every eight hours for two doses following surgery, and subsequently gradually reduced. Because postoperative irradiation was administered, she was given 20 mg hydrocortisone orally four times daily until this therapy was completed. She has subsequently been maintained on hydrocortisone, 7.5 mg four times daily, and there has been no evidence of recurrence of her cancer during the ensuing seven years. Menses tapered and stopped at age fifty-one. At age fifty-three her blood FSH was 121 mIU/ml, blood estrogen was 28.0 pg/ml, T_3 sponge uptake was 45 percent, and T_4 was 6.4 mcg%.* She has experienced moderately severe hot flashes and some arthritic symptoms but otherwise has felt well and is living a normal life.

This is an example of the occurrence of spontaneous Graves' disease, a known autoimmune disorder, and spontaneous adrenal insufficiency, a possible autoimmune disorder, in the same person. The history of irregular menstrual periods and infertility indicates some abnormality of the pituitary-ovarian axis, and the development of carcinoma in both breasts around the time of the menopause raises a question whether this disease might also be related in some way to her other endocrine abnormalities. In spite of these serious diagnoses, she has lived a

* Normal ranges for tests in Case Summaries are listed on p. 184.

relatively normal life for seven years following radical mastectomy. The increased incidence and severity of respiratory infections prior to treatment of her adrenal insufficiency contrasted with the increased resistance to such infections while taking cortisone acetate.

Case 3

This case is another example of spontaneous adrenal insufficiency that demonstrates the subtle relationship that exists between function of the adrenals, ovaries, and thyroid glands. The patient was referred at the age of twenty-eight years because of amenorrhea following discontinuance of an oral contraceptive. The menarche had occurred at age thirteen, and cycles had been regular at monthly intervals, menses lasting five to six days. She had been married at age twenty and had full-term Caesarean sections at ages twenty-one, twenty-two, and twenty-three years. She did not nurse any of her babies. After her third section she required a transfusion and experienced a transfusion reaction. Subsequently she felt chronically fatigued. After one spontaneous menstrual flow, she was given an oral contraceptive cyclically for about fifteen months. When this was discontinued spontaneous menses did not resume. Withdrawal bleeding occurred after various progestational agents. Occasional hot flashes were experienced, but she also was sensitive to cold. Her energy had continued to be poor. Salpingograms and a D. & C. had been reported normal. Her previous history had been negative except for a tonsillectomy at age six. Her mother had a total hysterectomy for an unknown cause at age thirty-four.

Physical examination was within normal limits with a height of 62 inches, weight 101½ pounds, blood pressure 95/70, and pulse 72 and regular. Urinary 17/KS were 1.5 mg/ 24 hours and urinary cortisol metabolites (similar to 17-OHST) were 2.3 mg/24 hours, both definitely low values. Urinary gonadotropins were within normal limits. After 80 units of ACTH gel intramuscularly, urinary 17-KS and cortisol metabolites did not change significantly, consistent with the presence of primary adrenal insufficiency. On hydrocortisone (Cortef®) 5 mg four times daily, she experienced marked symptomatic improvement and a resumption of spontaneous menses. These occurred at irregular intervals, however, so the dosage of Cortef was increased to 7.5 mg four times daily. Cycles were still irregular, so Euthroid®, gr. 1 daily, was added even though thyroid tests were within normal limits: T_3 index $= 0.91$ (normal 0.8-1.2), T_4 6.6 mcg% (normal 5.0-10.0). Serum cholesterol was slightly high, however, (266 mg%, with a normal range of 150-260 mg%), and she was sensitive to cold. On this program she conceived in 1972 and had a full-term Caesarean section nine months later. During her pregnancy she took hydrocortisone, 10 mg four times daily, and Euthroid, gr 1 daily. Her obstetrician had her discontinue the Euthroid in the eighth month.

After delivery, the patient received an injection to inhibit lactation, since she was not nursing her baby. Hydrocortisone was resumed in a dosage of 10 mg four times daily. She returned to my office four months later without having had any spontaneous menses, and she failed to have withdrawal flow after medroxyprogesterone acetate (Provera®), 5 mg daily for five days. The dosage of Cortef was decreased to 5 mg four times daily, and she resumed spontaneous menses about a month later, but her cycles were quite irregular.

Six months later an ACTH test revealed a baseline plasma cortisol at 10 AM of 21.5 mcg% (2½ hours after her last dose of 5 mg hydrocortisone), and an hour after an intramuscular (I.M.) injection of 25 units of ACTH, the plasma cortisol was 28.2 mcg%, consistent with persistent adrenal insufficiency.

The dosage of hydrocortisone was increased to 10 mg before breakfast and lunch, 5 mg before supper, and 10 mg at bedtime, with improvement in energy, but the patient read newspaper and magazine articles about the dangerous effects of cortisone therapy so she kept skipping doses and trying to wean herself off the medication. Each time she did this, she developed increased fatigue and malaise, so treatment was resumed. In 1976 another ACTH test performed with an I.M. injection of 25 units of Cortrosyn again failed to demonstrate an adrenal response. Plasma follicle-stimulating hormone (FSH) at that time was normal, but T_3 sponge uptake was 37 percent (normal 40-60%), and T_4, was 3.6 mcg% (normal 4.0-10.0). Because she had no symptoms of hypothyroidism, T_3 by RIA was measured, and this was 155 ng/100 ml, a value well within normal limits (90-200).

She therefore not only had adrenal insufficiency but also evidence of abnormal thyroid function characterized by a low T_3 sponge uptake and T_4 with a normal triiodothyronine level in the blood.

She failed to return for follow-up until two years later. During the previous year she had repeated respiratory infections and had become more sensitive to cold. T_3 sponge uptake was 35 percent, T_4 3.3, and T_3 by RIA had decreased to 20 ng/100 ml. The diagnosis of hypothyroidism was no longer in question, and Euthroid, gr 1 daily, was resumed with restoration of normal health and regular menses.

That this patient developed adrenal insufficiency after a transfusion reaction following her third Caesarean section raises a question of possible etiologic relationship. Could the transfusion reaction have initiated an autoimmune process that damaged her adrenals and possibly also her thyroid gland? She later developed post-contraceptive pill amenorrhea with normal FSH, and she resumed menses and conceived when replacement hydrocortisone and thyroid therapy were administered, subsequently having another full-term, normal pregnancy. Her obstetrician did not maintain communication with her endocrinologist during her pregnancy and delivery, and this may have affected her post partum course, since it is usually advisable for patients to continue physiologic dosages of hydrocortisone and thyroid up to the time of delivery, then resume these medications post partum in the dosages the patient was taking at the time she conceived.

The resumption of menses post partum was apparently affected by her replacement dosage of hydrocortisone and probably also by the cessation of thyroid medication. Post contraceptive amenorrhea is now known to be sometimes associated with an elevated level of plasma prolactin, but a test for it was not available at that time. She had no evidence of persistent lactation, however. Although she did not resume thyroid medication post partum, she did not develop definite clinical evidence of hypothyroidism until six years later, and her menstrual cycles did not become regular until thyroid replacement therapy was administered in addition to hydrocortisone. She is one of numerous patients who have become alarmed by literature that emphasizes the hazards of glucocorticoid therapy without mentioning that hydrocortisone is a natural hormone necessary for normal health and energy.

Case 4

This patient was totally adrenalectomized for Cushing's syndrome. The young woman was referred in 1967 at the age of twenty-four years with a chief complaint of rounding of her face and increased hair growth for the previous year. The menarche had occurred at age thirteen, and her cycles had always been irregular with intervals of thirty to sixty days, menses lasting five days without cramps. She had been married seven years previously and had a daughter six years old. She had had no difficulty conceiving and her pregnancy was normal. She did not nurse her baby, and menses resumed uneventfully.

Four impacted wisdom teeth had been removed at age twenty-one, and the patient thought her problems started after this dental surgery. For two years prior to her initial visit she had been more nervous, changed from being sensitive to cold to sensitive to heat, and developed diarrhea about once weekly. During the previous year she had noted more rounding of her face and some increased hair growth on her face. A gynecologist had performed a wedge resection of her ovaries 6 months before her visit. The ovaries were said to be only slightly enlarged, but bilateral cysts were present. Her menses continued to be irregular. Her weight had increased from 115 to 122 pounds over the previous year. Her mother and maternal grandmother had had thyroid operations, and her maternal grandmother also had diabetes mellitus. There was no family history of hypertension.

Physical examination revealed a young woman with definite rounding of the face and moderate hirsutism of the face and periareolar areas. Height was 63¼ inches, weight was 122 pounds without shoes. Mild acne was present on the shoulders and back, but there were no striae. Blood pressure was 165/105, pulse 96 and regular. The thyroid was not enlarged, and there was no lymphadenopathy. Breast development was normal with slight deep induration on the right. There was no edema, and no bruises were present. The remainder of her examination was not remarkable. Plasma cortisol at 8 AM was 23.0 and at 4 PM was 31.8 mcg%. Urinary 17-KS were 19.6 and cortisol metabolites 22.5 mg/ 24 hours. A brisk response to ACTH stimulation occurred, and dexamethasone suppressed plasma cortisol and urinary 17-KS and cortisol metabolites to normal. An x-ray of the skull showed no enlargement of the sella turcica. A diagnosis of Cushing's syndrome with adrenal hyperplasia was therefore made.

She was given sufficient dexamethasone to keep her steroid levels normal, but her adrenals continued to become hyperactive whenever the dosage of dexamethasone was decreased, and cushingoid features worsened while she was taking this medication. A total bilateral adrenalectomy was therefore performed. Postoperatively she was maintained on hydrocortisone, 10 mg four times daily, and 9-α-FF, 0.1 mg three times weekly. After surgery her blood pressure became normal but gradually increased from 130/85 to 140/100, so the 9-α-FF was tapered and discontinued. Hydrodiuril®, 50 mg daily, and later Inderal®, 10 mg four times daily, caused the blood pressure to decrease to 125/90. After approximately a year, the hydrochlorathiazide was discontinued without significantly affecting the blood pressure, and later Inderal was discontinued. For the past three years her blood pressure has varied between 120 and 140/80 to 100/ with no antihypertensive medication.

In spite of her maintenance therapy the patient continued to complain of chronic fatigue, so a month after adrenalectomy dehydroepiandrosterone (DHA), 5 mg by mouth twice daily, was started. A limited supply of this steroid had been provided by Ayerst Laboratories for clinical investigation. This produced impressive improvement in her energy, and she developed spontaneous menses at monthly intervals, the first time she had ever had regular menstrual cycles. Because our supply of DHA was limited, it was discontinued after she had achieved optimum clinical improvement on four different occasions, and each time she developed a return of fatigue and irregular menses, sometimes associated with functional bleeding, and she also noted that she bruised more easily when she was not taking this steroid.

When it was resumed, energy improved, menstrual cycles became regular, and she no longer bruised easily. Other androgens, including methyl testosterone, Halotestin®, and testosterone propionate, were tried, but none of these restored normal menses or produced as much improvement in energy as the DHA. Vitamin C, 100 mg daily, was also tried, but it did not produce the clinical improvement noted with DHA.

Follow-up skull x-rays were normal. Five years after adrenalectomy her pigmentation, which had increased initially, appeared to be definitely subsiding. Urinary FSH was 10 mouse uterine units (m.u.u.) and total estrogens 29 μg/24 hours, both within normal limits for a female. She was not taking DHA at the time of these tests. Six years postadrenalectomy plasma ACTH by RIA was 49.9 pg/ml (normal 15-100). Six years ago her medication was changed from hydrocortisone to cortisone acetate, 10 mg before breakfast, before lunch, and at bedtime, and 5 mg before supper, and she thought this caused less tendency to indigestion.

In October, 1975, our supply of DHA was exhausted, and shortly after that her menses ceased and she noted increased fatigue. Methyl testosterone, one 5 mg linguet daily, was administered with some improvement in energy, but amenorrhea has persisted. We have not yet been able to obtain an additional supply of DHA for clinical investigation.

This patient has been followed for thirteen years after a total bilateral adrenalectomy for Cushing's syndrome. Although she has done fairly well, the evidence was convincing that DHA provided an improvement in energy and a resumption of normal menstrual cycles that was not matched by any other androgen. It was also our impression that DHA caused her to bruise less easily. Andrews[9] has reviewed the experimental evidence for possible mechanisms of reproductive suppression by increased ACTH secretion, but it also appears that a deficient production of DHA may have a similar effect. Some patients with Cushing's syndrome have been reported to develop progressive enlargement of pituitary adenomas after adrenalectomy, but there has been no evidence of such a problem in this patient, and the question arises whether such developments might be related to a suboptimum schedule of replacement therapy.

LOW ADRENAL RESERVE

As mentioned previously, low adrenal reserve is another clinical disorder in which physiologic dosages of cortisone or hydrocortisone have a rational role in therapy. This is a condition in which baseline levels of hydrocortisone in the plasma are within normal limits, but patients are unable to respond to stress with an adequate increase in production of hydrocortisone by their adrenals. It is diagnosed by subnormal response to ACTH with a normal baseline plasma cortisol level.

An impressive number of patients with chronic fatigue have been found to have low adrenal reserve, and the administration of cortisone acetate or hydrocortisone in dosages of 5 mg four times daily has resulted in clinical improvement that is often dramatic. Because of the residual adrenal tissue, the bedtime dosage may be omitted in such patients, permitting a more normal diurnal variation in plasma cortisol levels. Most of these patients have been studied intensively prior to being referred for endocrine evaluation, receiving various other types of therapy, including vitamins, iron, and thyroid medication, without benefit. That many had been told their fatigue must have a psychogenic basis when previous studies had failed to demonstrate any evidence of organic disorder emphasizes the importance of this condition.

Patients with psychiatric disorders, especially depression, frequently complain of chronic fatigue, but their adrenals characteristically are hyperresponsive to ACTH,[10, 11] so an ACTH test should distinguish them from patients with low adrenal reserve. Patients with low adrenal reserve describe wanting to do things but feeling too exhausted to undertake them, and they usually present no evidence of serious psychologic problems. Another helpful diagnostic point is that patients with low adrenal reserve typically describe a type of fatigue that is present throughout the day, often being noted when they first awaken in the morning, in contrast to the fatigue that is present in patients with hypothyroidism, which characteristically does not develop until afternoon or evening. Patients with known psychologic problems who complain of fatigue should also have ACTH tests, because in some cases it appears that the chronic fatigue resulting from low adrenal reserve has aggravated a psychic disorder, and if the chronic fatigue can be helped, the psychologic disorder may also be benefited.

Patients with functional hypoglycemia should also have ACTH tests because, as is discussed later (Chapter 10), almost all of the patients referred with this diagnosis have been found to have low adrenal reserve. This is not surprising in view of the function of glucocorticoids in preventing hypoglycemia.

Many patients with allergic disorders such as bronchial asthma or allergic rhinitis also complain of chronic fatigue, and about half of them have been found to have abnormal ACTH tests, with evidence of either low adrenal reserve or of a low baseline level of plasma cortisol. Low adrenal reserve suggests some primary disorder in adrenocortical function, whereas a low baseline level of plasma cortisol with a normal response to ACTH suggests a mild deficiency in the hypothalamus or pituitary or a low corticosteroid-binding protein. This will be discussed further in Chapter 7.

The etiology of low adrenal reserve is not known, but it is interesting to note that heavy cigarette smoking[12] and ingestion of moderate amounts of coffee[13] have been found to cause significant rises in plasma and urinary 11-hydroxycorticosteroid concentrations, possibly due to enhanced ACTH release resulting from nicotine — or caffeine — induced increases in sympathetic and catecholamine activity. Whether prolonged adrenocortical stimulation from these or other causes could result in low adrenal reserve in susceptible persons remains speculative.

The possibility that ascorbic acid deficiency might cause low adrenal reserve should also be studied. The highest concentration of ascorbic acid in the body occurs in the adrenal cortex, but its function there has never been elucidated. Presumably it plays a role in the production of adrenocortical steroids. Administration of large dosages of vitamin C has been reported to have a protective effect against the common cold as well as some other beneficial effects that have been noted with physiologic dosages of cortisone or hydrocortisone,[14] so a relationship would not be surprising.

It should be emphasized that clinical improvement from physiologic dosages of cortisone or hydrocortisone may not become evident for up to two weeks after the initiation of this therapeutic program, so patients should be cautioned not to become discouraged if they do not feel better immediately.

It is not advised that all patients with unexplained fatigue be given glucocorticoids, but further studies to determine the nature of possible adrenal or pituitary dysfunction in such cases, as well as careful allergic work-ups, are encouraged. The interference with normal daily living described by such patients is sufficient to warrant careful investigation, especially since the chances of restoring energy and a sense of well-being seem to be quite good.

Several case histories provide examples of the value of this type of therapy in patients with low adrenal reserve.

Case 5

The patient was a fifty-six year old female who had experienced episodes of nausea and fainting for approximately twenty years. At first these episodes would occur at intervals of one or two years, but at about age fifty-four they became more frequent, as often as once a week. They were usually associated with headache. At age fifty-four she was admitted to a hospital where a neurological consultation reported no evidence of abnormality, but blood sugar was noted to be low three hours after glucose administration during a routine glucose tolerance test. X-rays of the skull, and brain and liver scans were all normal, and she was discharged with a diagnosis of functional hypoglycemia.

After discharge she experienced little benefit from dietary therapy and began to complain of chronic fatigue as well, so at age fifty-six she was referred for an endocrinologic evaluation. Because she was receiving medications including Dilantin®, Bellergal®, and Pro-Banthine®, some of which might interfere with plasma cortisol determinations, and because her symptoms were somewhat suggestive of adrenal insufficiency, she was given a therapeutic trial with hydrocortisone, 5 mg four times daily.

She returned two weeks later reporting dramatic improvement. She was, therefore, tapered off of all medications. A week after discontinuing hydrocortisone, her plasma cortisol at 9 AM was 19.3 mcg%, and one hour after an I.M. injection of 25 units of ACTH this rose to 38.2 mcg%, a response at the lower range of normal. She developed weakness and fatigue off the medication, however, so hydrocortisone was again resumed in a dosage of 5 mg four times daily, with another impressive subjective response.

It was therefore decided to obtain a metopirone test to check on the possibility of hypopituitarism causing her symptoms, but this test also was within normal limits. Hydrocortisone had been discontinued the day before the metopirone test was started. She was then instructed to discontinue the hydrocortisone for six weeks, following which a second ACTH test showed very clear evidence of low adrenal reserve, with a baseline plasma cortisol level of 21.7 mcg% at 9 AM and a rise to only 26.7 mcg% after ACTH. Meanwhile, she had again developed symptoms of frequent headaches, nausea, chronic fatigue, and malaise. She again improved after the resumption of hydrocortisone, 5 mg four times daily.

The patient still tired somewhat easily, however, and when she developed an upper respiratory infection and her dosage was increased to 10 mg four times daily, she stated she felt so much better that her maintenance dosage was increased to 7.5 mg four times daily. She has continued to feel quite well on this dosage. She has now received this therapy for a total of five years, during which time she has had no undesirable side effects and has felt better than she had for many years. She has experienced several respiratory infections, but when her dosage was doubled, she recovered promptly. On two occasions she has been given penicillin and on two occasions erythromycin for sinusitis during the past five years.

This case demonstrates how unexplained nausea and faintness, especially when associated with functional hypoglycemia, should suggest the possibility of adrenal insufficiency or low adrenal reserve. It also demonstrates how therapy with glucocorticoid can result in a temporary restoration of adrenal reserve that may relapse after glucocorticoid is withheld for several weeks. In addition, she provides an example of how respiratory infections can be well tolerated with the therapeutic glucocorticoid program recommended.

Case 6

This patient was a fifty-one year old female. She had reached the menarche at age fourteen with regular cycles at intervals of twenty-eight days until she went to college, when menses ceased. They resumed at the time of spring and summer vacations, however, consistent with a diagnosis of "psychogenic amenorrhea." She was married at age twenty-two, used no precautions, but was unable to conceive. Her husband was found to have a low sperm count, so they adopted two children.

At age forty the patient had operations for bilateral inguinal hernias, and the surgeon noted the presence of endometriosis, so a few months later a hysterectomy and bilateral salpingo-oophorectomy were performed. She was given Premarin, 0.625 mg daily on a cyclic schedule, but hot flashes persisted, so the dosage was increased to 1.25 mg cyclically. This corrected the hot flashes, but she developed intermittent stiffness and aching in the knees and other joints, and she tended to tire more easily.

For several years the patient had noted numbness in her hands and toes after exposure to cold and after sleeping, and this became worse. Her skin tended to be dry, and she had mild constipation. T_3 sponge uptake and serum thyroxine were normal, but an ACTH test revealed low adrenal reserve with a baseline plasma cortisol of 19.4 mcg% at 9 AM and a rise to 25.9 mcg% thirty minutes after an I.M. injection of Cortrosyn. Hydrocortisone, 5 mg four times daily, was started, and within two weeks she noted marked subjective improvement with normal energy, disappearance of arthralgias, and a general increase in sense of well-being. Cyclic Premarin therapy was maintained.

The patient continued to feel well over the subsequent five years and has reported increased resistance to respiratory infections. Whenever symptoms of incipient respiratory infections have developed, the dosage of hydrocortisone has been doubled until the symptoms cleared. On several occasions symptoms have disappeared within twenty-four hours with such therapy, suggesting that the illness had been aborted. During this time her husband had numerous respiratory infections, so there has been no apparent change in her exposure to such infections.

In this patient low adrenal reserve was initially manifested by intermittent arthritic symptoms as well as chronic fatigue following a surgical menopause. This condition has been termed "menopausal arthritis," and this patient's experience indicates the advisability of testing adrenal responsiveness in such patients. Improvement with small physiologic dosages of cortisone acetate or hydrocortisone may be dramatic. It is tempting to speculate that the "psychogenic amenorrhea" was a manifestation of mild adrenocortical dysfunction, the increased stress of attending college causing excessive adrenal production of estrogen, which in turn caused amenorrhea. Later, after bilateral herniorrhaphy and bilateral salpingo-oophorectomy, the increased demand upon the adrenals may have resulted in symptoms of fatigue and arthritis that were corrected by hydrocortisone administration. Cyclic Premarin therapy was continued because she had not yet reached the usual age of spontaneous menopause. She has had no further symptoms of endometriosis. She is one of numerous patients who have reported evidence of increased resistance to respiratory infections while taking small doses of cortisone acetate or hydrocortisone, and this will be discussed in more detail in Chapter 9.

Another example of low adrenal reserve is presented in case number 7.

Case 7

A fifty-nine year old female had been experiencing episodes of fatigue since the age of forty-six. Her menstrual history had been normal until age thirty-five, when she developed prolonged uterine bleeding. Radium therapy to the endometrium had been administered for this, and she developed subsequent amenorrhea and hot flashes. The episodes of fatigue began about ten years later. Her previous physician had given her dexamethasone for four days empirically with suggestive benefit. Later, when her symptoms returned, she had been given various other medications, including estrogen and androgens, without apparent effect. She had also been given thyroid medication without benefit. Four months prior to her referral, she had been given prednisone, 5 mg twice daily with dramatic improvement, but when the dosage was reduced to 5 mg daily, fatigue returned. She was therefore referred as a possible case of adrenal insufficiency.

Because the patient had been taking prednisone, an ACTH test was not performed initially, but her medication was changed to hydrocortisone in decreasing dosages. It was found that she felt best on a dosage of 7.5 mg four times daily. While receiving that dosage she had an ACTH test that demonstrated a plasma cortisol at 10 AM of 13.7 mcg%; one hour after an I.M. injection of 25 units of ACTH this rose to 22.9 mcg%, consistent with a sluggish adrenal response. She has subsequently felt quite well on 7.5 mg four times daily. On several occasions when the dosage was decreased to 5 mg four times daily, fatigue returned, and various aches developed, especially in her shoulders and neck.

In 1975 a return of chronic fatigue occurred while the patient was taking hydrocortisone, 7.5 mg four times daily, and it was found that she had an infected tooth. Energy returned when the dental infection was treated. She gave a history of having never had upper respiratory infections or influenza during her lifetime, nor has she had any incidence of these infections since she has been taking hydrocortisone. She had had two episodes of urinary tract infection, but these responded promptly to cephalosporin therapy. A year ago she had an uneventful vaginal repair of a rectocele and enterocele with a perineorrhaphy, receiving additional hydrocortisone prior to and following her surgery. An ACTH test performed during her hospitalization showed persistent low adrenal reserve.

This is another patient who had developed symptoms of fatigue in her mid forties, which ultimately proved to be due to low adrenal reserve. She had experienced menopause following pelvic irradiation ten years previously. She also noted various aches and arthritic symptoms associated with chronic fatigue, and all of these symptoms were corrected by suitable physiologic dosages of hydrocortisone. Later, the return of symptoms while she was taking hydrocortisone was found to be due to the development of a dental infection, emphasizing the importance of looking for obscure infections in patients who have a relapse of symptoms while taking a dosage of steroid that has previously been sufficient to control their condition. This patient is also one of several patients whom we have encountered who give a history of never having had respiratory infections or influenza, suggesting the presence of an immune mechanism that provides greater than usual resistance to this type of illness. Her case is another example of how patients with adrenal insufficiency or low reserve can tolerate elective surgery uneventfully provided they are given additional hydrocortisone prior to and following the stress.

CONGENITAL ADRENAL HYPERPLASIA

Another disorder in which treatment with physiologic dosages of cortisone or hydrocortisone is obviously indicated is congenital adrenal hyperplasia. This condition results from a relative deficiency of one of the enzymes in the pathway of production of hydrocortisone in the adrenals. The deficiency in hydrocortisone production leads to increased ACTH stimulation that in turn causes an excessive production of those steroids that do not require the deficient enzyme. The most common defect is in 21-hydroxylase, the enzyme that converts 17-alpha-hydroxyprogesterone to cortexolone. This deficiency is usually relative rather than absolute so that the adrenals produce an excess of androgen and other steroids that do not require this enzyme to supply sufficient hydrocortisone. The clinical picture is most obvious in young girls who, as a result of androgen excess, have abnormal development of the genitalia with enlargement of the clitoris, rapid skeletal growth in early childhood but premature closure of the epiphyses, resulting in ultimate short stature, androgenic build, acne, hirsutism, and poor secondary sexual development with amenorrhea and hypoplasia of the breasts.

Treatment of the disorder consists of the administration of sufficient cortisone acetate or hydrocortisone to reduce the excessive levels of androgen and ACTH to normal. The maximum maintenance level for the unstressed patient should therefore be 35-40 mg daily of either cortisone acetate or hydrocortisone, and many patients can be maintained on smaller dosages. Earlier reports suggested that larger doses might be necessary, but this was probably due to a suboptimum dosage schedule. Although these patients usually tolerate stress without developing adrenal insufficiency, they should be instructed to increase the dosages with stress in a manner similar to patients with adrenal insufficiency so as to avoid an excessive production of androgen during the stress.

With suitable therapy patients with congenital adrenal hyperplasia will develop normally and be able to bear children provided treatment is instituted early and taken regularly in an optimum dosage. Even when treatment is started later in life, improvement is usually impressive, but fertility is less predictable. The schedule of dividing the daily dosage into four equal doses to be taken with meals and at bedtime provides a more effective suppression of excessive androgen production than a schedule of only two doses daily (Fig 4).[15]

Because 21-hydroxylase is also necessary for the production of sodium-retaining steroids, there is no excess of these steroids in 21-hydroxylase deficiency. In a less common type of congenital adrenal hyperplasia due to a relative deficiency of 11-beta-hydroxylase, an excess of the sodium-retaining steroid 11-desoxycorticosterone as well as of androgens occurs, and the patients have hypertension associated with androgenicity. The pathologic physiology is still essentially the same — the adrenals are being stimulated to work overtime to produce a sufficient supply of hydrocortisone, and in the process they produce an excess of other steroids. Hence, the treatment is the same: administration of sufficient hydrocortisone to restore normal levels of the other steroids. In patients with 11-beta-hydroxylase deficiency, treatment with hydrocortisone not only counteracts the androgenicity but also restores blood pressure to normal, provided permanent damage to the kidneys has not occurred. These patients have an interesting combination of relative

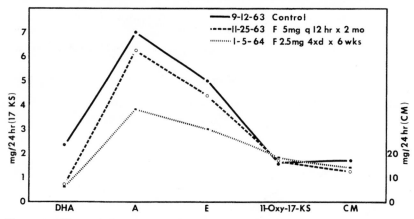

Figure 4. Effects of the same total daily dosage of hydrocortisone administered in 2 divided doses and in 4 divided doses. F = hydrocortisone, DHA = dehydroepiandrosterone, A = androsterone, E = etiocholanolone, 11-oxy-17-KS = 11-oxygenated 17 ketosteroids, and CM = cortisol metabolites. The values for fractions from each separate 24-hour urine collection are connected by lines to facilitate comparison. From William McK Jefferies, Glucocorticoids and Ovulation, in RB Greenblatt (Ed.), *Ovulation.* Copyright 1966, J. B. Lippincott Co., Philadelphia. Reprinted by permission.

adrenal insufficiency with hypertension and emphasize that a low blood pressure is not essential for the diagnosis of relative adrenal insufficiency.

A patient who demonstrates the subtle aspects of diagnosing this type of congenital adrenal hyperplasia is described in case 8.

Case 8

This forty-three year old male was referred because of recurrent hyperthyroidism. He had had high blood pressure as long as he could remember, but he did not know what treatment he had been given for this. He had not been taking any medication for several months prior to his visit. He said he was a large baby at birth and that he had been very strong as a child. He remembered eating heartily when he was three years old, and he was unusually strong until age eighteen, when his strength seemed to leave him suddenly, about the time he had a tumor removed from his right breast. Symptoms of hyperthyroidism had developed at age thirty-seven; he took medication for this for two years with improvement.

A year before his referral, at age forty-two, he had a return of nervousness that he attributed to a vasectomy that had been performed four months previously. Six months later he had influenza and was quite ill with complicating pneumonia. Subsequently his symptoms of excessive nervousness and fatigue became worse. He had felt warm and had noted an increased pulse rate, but there had been no change in weight. Prior to the influenza attack, he said he had had no respiratory infection for at least ten years.

The patient denied having ever had any headaches, but his energy had frequently been poor. He was married and had three children. There was no family history of diabetes mellitus, but his mother had high blood pressure.

Physical examination revealed a height of 65½ inches, weight 152½ pounds, blood pressure 160-170/90-100, pulse 88 and regular. He was very tense and restless, with moderate hirsutism. There were no eye signs of hyperthyroidism and he had minimal tremor. The thyroid was soft, difficult to outline, approximately two-and-one-half times normal size. There was no lymphadenopathy. The remainder of his examination was not remarkable. White blood count was 5,900 with 76 percent neutrophils, 22 percent lymphs, 1 percent monocytes, and 1 percent eosinophils. Twenty-four hour I^{131} uptake over the thyroid was 29 percent; T_3 sponge uptake was 67 percent (normal 40-60 percent), and T_4 was 9.4 mcg% (normal 4.0-10.0). T_3 by RIA was 180 mcg% (normal 65-215). Plasma cortisol at 1:15 PM was 10.9 µg%, a relatively low value for this time of day, but thirty minutes after an I.M. injection of 25 units of Cortrosyn this rose to 27.9 µg%, consistent with normal adrenal responsiveness.

Because his history suggested the presence of excessive androgen at an early age plus asymptomatic hypertension for many years, a blood sample was drawn for plasma desoxycorticosterone. This was reported to be 355 ng%, with a normal range of 5-15. Repeat determinations obtained several weeks later were 275 and 349 ng%.

This patient therefore had not only symptoms suggestive of a mild recurrence of hyperthyroidism without laboratory confirmation but also congenital adrenal hyperplasia characterized by excessive production of androgen and desoxycorticosterone. A diagnosis of congenital adrenal hyperplasia associated with a deficiency of 11-beta-hydroxylase was therefore made. Hydrocortisone, 5 mg four times daily, was prescribed, and his strength and sense of well-being improved impressively, but symptoms of hyperthyroidism became more pronounced; T_4 increased to 12.5 mcg% and T_3 by RIA to 250 ng/100 ml, so propylthiouracil, 50 mg four times daily, was added to his therapy. T_3 and T_4 and symptoms of hyperthyroidism returned to normal, but plasma desoxycorticosterone remained elevated until the dosage of hydrocortisone was increased to 7.5 mg four times daily. Five months later T_3 by RIA was 160 ng/100 ml, T_4 9.0 mcg%, and plasma desoxycorticosterone 6.8 ng/100 ml. Blood pressure decreased to 120-135/80-90. It was therefore evident that he not only experienced symptomatic improvement on hydrocortisone therapy but blood pressure also decreased to normal range. Propylthiouracil was discontinued after a year, and hyperthyroidism has remained in remission.

The recurrence of hyperthyroidism with a diffuse thyroid enlargement in this patient with congenital adrenal hyperplasia, and the apparent aggravation of symptoms and laboratory evidence of hyperthyroidism after the patient received hydrocortisone, raise a question of the possible significance of adrenocortical function in patients developing hyperthyroidism. That Graves' disease, or hyperthyroidism due to diffuse goiter, has been demonstrated to be a manifestation of an autoimmune phenomenon associated with the production of an abnormal thyroid stimulator, and the apparent relationship between autoimmune phenomena and adrenocortical function, provide support for such speculation. In addition, evidence that physiologic dosages of hydrocortisone may increase T_3 receptor function, as discussed in Chapter 10, further suggests a possible mechanism of the influence of hydrocortisone upon thyroid function. A deficiency of 11-beta-hydroxylase is thought to be a relatively rare cause of hypertension, but it should be considered in women with hypertension plus associated androgenic changes or elevated urinary 17-KS and in hypertensive men, especially in younger age groups. Perhaps it may be more common than is presently suspected. It is interesting to note that an earlier report[16] mentioned a blood pressure lowering effect of cortisone as well as a blood pressure elevating effect of ACTH in some hypertensives. The occurrence of partial 11- and 21-hydroxylase deficiencies in patients who develop hypertension, hirsutism, and menstrual disorders in late childhood or early adulthood[17, 18, 19] has been demonstrated and termed "acquired" adrenal hyperplasia, emphasizing the importance of careful studies in such cases. An interesting feature of hypertension associated with 11-beta-hydroxylase deficiency is that it may persist for years without complications such as renal damage. The ability to test for elevated levels of desoxycorticosterone in blood or urine should simplify the diagnosis of this curable form of hypertension.

REFERENCES

1. Irvine WJ, Barnes EW: In Gell PGH, Coombs RRA, Lachman PJ, (Eds.): *Clinical Aspects of Immunology,* 3rd ed. Oxford, Blackwells, 1975, pp. 1301-1354.
2. Wood JB, Frankland AW, James VHT, Landon J: A rapid test of adrenocortical function, *Lancet 1:*243-245, 1965.
3. Greig WR, Maxwell JD, Boyle JA, Lindsay RM, Browning McK: Criteria for distinguishing normal from subnormal adrenocortical function using the synacthen test. *Postgrad Med J 45:*307-313, 1969.
4. Barnes ND, Joseph HM, Atherdem SM, Clayton BE: Functional tests of adrenal axis in children with measurement of plasma cortisol by competitive protein-binding. *Arch Dis Child 47:*66-73, 1972.
5. Liddle GW: The adrenal cortex. In Williams RH (Ed.): *Textbook of Endocrinology.* Philadelphia, Saunders, 1974, p. 275.
6. Jefferies WMcK, Kelly LW, Sydnor KL, Levy RP, Cooper G: Metabolic effects of a single intravenous infusion of hydrocortisone related to plasma levels in a normal versus an adrenally insufficient subject. *J Clin Endocrinol Metab 17:*186-200, 1957.
7. Zetzel L: The use of ACTH and adrenocorticosteroids in diseases of the digestive system. *N Engl J Med 257:*1170-1180, 1957.
8. Jefferies WMcK: Low dosage glucocorticoid therapy. *Arch Intern Med 119:*265-278, 1967.
9. Andrews RV: Influence of the adrenal gland on gonadal function. In Thomas JA, Singhal RL (Eds.): *Advances in Sex Hormone Research, Vol. 3: Regulatory Mechanisms Affecting Gonadal Hormone Action,* Baltimore, Univ Park, 1976, pp. 197-215.
10. Altschule MD, Promisel E, Parkhurst BH, Grunebaum H: Effects of ACTH in patients with mental disease. *Arch Neurol Psychiatry 64:*641-649, 1950.
11. Elithorn A, Bridges PK, Hodges JR, Jones MT: Adrenocortical responsiveness during courses of electro-convulsive therapy. *Br J Psychiatry 115:*575-580, 1969.
12. Kershbaum A, Pappajohn DJ, Bellet S, Hirabayashi M, Shafiiha A: Effect of smoking and nicotine on adrenocortical secretion. *JAMA 203:*275-278, 1968.
13. Bellet S, Kostis J, Roman L, DeCastro O: Effect of coffee ingestion on adrenocortical secretion in young men and dogs. *Metabolism 18:*1007-1012, 1969.
14. Pauling L: *Vitamin C, the Common Cold and Flu.* San Francisco, Freeman, 1976.
15. Jefferies WMcK: Glucocorticoids and ovulation. In Greenblatt, RB (Ed.): *Ovulation.* Philadelphia, Lippincott, 1966, pp. 62-74.
16. Perera GA: In Mote JR (Ed.): *Proceedings of the First Clinical ACTH Conference.* Philadelphia, Blakiston, 1950, p. 284.

17. Gabrilove JL, Sharma DC, Dorfman RJ: Adrenocortical 11β-hydroxylase deficiency and virilism first manifest in the adult woman. *N Engl J Med* *272:*1189-1194, 1965.

18. Newmark S, Dluhy RG, Williams GH, Pochi P, Rose LI: Partial 11-and 21-hydroxylase deficiencies in hirsute women. *Am J Obstet Gynecol* *127:*594-598, 1977.

19. Tan SY, Noth RH, Mulrow PJ: Deoxycorticosterone and 17-ketosteroids: Elevated levels in hypertensive patients. *JMAG 240:*123-126, 1978.

Chapter 5

GONADAL DYSFUNCTION

THE BENEFICIAL EFFECTS of physiologic dosages of cortisone acetate and hydrocortisone in patients with congenital adrenal hyperplasia led to their being tried in women with ovarian dysfunction, hirsutism, and acne, since this combination of abnormalities occurred in both types of conditions. The dosages of glucocorticoids initially administered were relatively large, in the range of the full replacement dosages employed in congenital adrenal hyperplasia. Improvement occurred, but the possibility of adrenocortical suppression and impairment of resistance to stress from such doses was disturbing, so progressively smaller doses were tried, and we were pleased to find that impressive improvement occurred from physiologic dosages of 5 mg four times daily or even 2.5 mg four times daily, provided treatment was continued for a sufficient length of time.[1] It was therefore postulated that such cases might represent variants of the adrenogenital syndrome, viz., mild disorders of adrenal steroid metabolism characterized by excessive production of adrenal androgen and estrogen in sufficient quantities to interfere with ovarian function.

At that time, assessment of adrenal steroid production was limited clinically to measurements of urinary excretion of 17-ketosteroids (17-KS) and 17-hydroxycorticosteroids (17-OHST), resulting in indirect estimates at best, since levels of urinary metabolites might be affected by steroid metabolism in the liver and peripheral tissues, by blood levels of steroid-binding proteins, or by renal function, as well as by changes in rate or pattern of steroid production by the adrenals.

Responses of urinary excretion of 17-KS and 17-OHST of these patients to a standard stimulus with ACTH were usually consistent with normal adrenal responsiveness, but when urinary 17-KS were fractionated, excretion of dehydroepiandrosterone (DHA), androsterone (A), and etiocholanolone (E) frequently showed much greater variation than that of women with regular ovulatory cycles.[2]

Later, when plasma levels of cortisol, testosterone, DHA-sulfate, estrogen, and FSH could be measured, it was found that some women with gonadal dysfunction that could be corrected by subreplacement dosages of cortisone acetate or hydrocortisone had poor responsiveness to ACTH indicative of low adrenal reserve, some had elevated levels of free (or unbound) testosterone or of DHA-sulfate, and some had elevated or low levels of estrogen and low or normal levels of FSH. Those with elevated plasma free testosterone had associated acne and hirsutism, but urinary 17-KS excretion might be within normal limits. On the other hand, some women with acne and/or hirsutism might have normal plasma testosterone with elevated urinary 17-ketosteroids, indicating the production of an excess of androgen other than testosterone, usually DHA-sulfate. Women with elevated levels of estrogen usually had metropathia hemorrhagica.

After subreplacement dosages of glucocorticoids were found to correct ovarian dysfunction in this type of patient, studies were undertaken to determine the effects of small doses of cortisone acetate on fluid and electrolyte excretion as well as urinary steroid levels.[3] It was found that small changes in urinary sodium and potassium excretion did occur but that these changes were corrected within eight days even though the steroid was continued (*see* Fig. 2). It was also noted that a new, stable level of urinary steroid excretion did not occur until approximately ten to fourteen days after these small doses were initiated. It was further found that these small doses did not interfere with the adrenals' ability to respond to a standard dose of ACTH[3] (Fig. 5).

The concept of a close functional relationship between the ovaries and the adrenals is not new. The steroid-forming tissues of the gonads and adrenal cortices have a common embryonic origin, and these glands share many enzymatic steps in the production of their steroid hormones. The changes in adrenocortical activity that occur at puberty and the menopause further suggest a close association between these two pairs of glands. The well-known effects of stress upon the function of both of

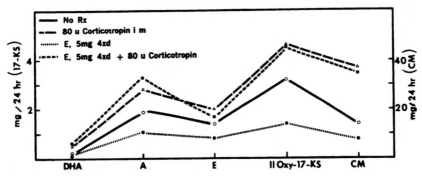

Figure 5. Effects of same dose of corticotropin administered to a 13 year old girl with probable rheumatoid arthritis upon urinary steroid fractions before treatment and while in a symptomatic remission on cortisone acetate (E), 5 mg 4 times daily (4xd). From William McK Jefferies, Low Dosage Glucocorticoid Therapy, *Archives of Internal Medicine*, 119:265-278. Copyright 1967, the American Medical Association. Reprinted by permission.

these pairs of glands could be due to simultaneous independent effects or to a sequential effect wherein the effect of stress upon one pair of glands, e.g. the adrenals, in turn affected the function of the other pair of glands. Clinical observations that patients with disorders of adrenocortical function, such as adrenal insufficiency (Addison's disease), hyperfunction (Cushing's syndrome), or dysfunction (congenital adrenal hyperplasia), had associated disorders of gonadal function were consistent with the concept of a close relationship between these glands. Furthermore, when cortisone was first tried in women with rheumatoid arthritis, interference with normal menstrual cycles was reported.[4, 5]

In spite of such abundant suggestive evidence of a functional relationship between the gonads and adrenal cortices, this relationship has not been very intensively studied. Andrews[6] has summarized reports prior to 1976 relative to this relationship and pointed out the need for more work in this field. The work of Kitay and his associates[7, 8] emphasizes the subtle nature but important potential of these relationships. They found that in castrated rats estrogen replacement increases ACTH secretion and decreases adrenal responsiveness to ACTH, whereas androgen decreases ACTH and increases adrenal responsiveness to ACTH. They also reported that low doses of testosterone stimulate adrenal enzymatic and steroidogenic capacity, but large doses have inhibitory effects. Furthermore, testosterone may potentiate the action of ACTH.[9] The possible effects of adrenal progesterone upon gonadal function remain to be clarified.

Our observations in women with adrenal insufficiency reported in Chapter 4 also indicate the sensitive but potent interactions of these two sets of glands. The occurrence of amenorrhea in these women, the restoration of normal menstrual cycles and fertility by administration of physiologic dosages of cortisone acetate or hydrocortisone in cases of spontaneous deficiency, and the requirement for supplementary small doses of dehydroepiandrosterone in the patient with total bilateral adrenalectomy exemplify this relationship.

Initially treatment of ovarian dysfunction with small dosages of cortisone acetate or hydrocortisone was restricted to patients with associated acne or hirsutism, but after observing the safety and beneficial effects of such therapy, it was decided to try similar dosages on patients who had ovarian dysfunction without hirsutism or acne. Many of these patients also experienced improvement in their clinical disorders.

Menstrual problems encountered included amenorrhea, either primary or secondary, but more often the latter, irregular menses, functional uterine bleeding, and luteal phase disorders. Women with ovarian dysfunction tend to have a high rate of infertility; small doses of cortisone acetate or hydrocortisone not only resulted in improvement of abnormal menstrual cycles but also in ability to conceive and to carry pregnancies normally to term. Effective dosages were as small as 2.5 mg every eight hours but usually were 2.5 or 5 mg four times daily.[10-13] Because these dosages do not impair resistance to stress, it is not necessary to give additional glucocorticoid at delivery, even if Caesarean section is performed, unless the patient had evidence of low adrenal reserve prior to treatment. Because the dosages are physiologic, they may be continued during lactation without harm to either the mother or her infant.

These findings were initially reported in 1958,[1] but meanwhile reports of harmful side effects of large doses of glucocorticoids were becoming so frequent that any dosage was viewed with alarm. By the time that I was able to report results on a significant series of cases,[14] patents had expired on cortisone acetate and hydrocortisone, and there was no incentive for pharmaceutical houses to seek further clinical uses of these agents even though the results of this therapy were impressive. Over 80 percent of women with ovarian dysfunction not related to some other disorder such as pituitary insufficiency or primary ovarian deficiency experienced a restoration of normal menstrual cycles, and of those who had associated fertility problems, 62 percent conceived and carried their pregnancies normally to term, provided they continued to take the medication throughout the pregnancy.

Meanwhile, clomiphene sulfate had been introduced as an agent to help stimulate ovulation and promote fertility in patients experiencing difficulty in conceiving. Clomiphene is not a natural hormone, but it is effective in some patients, and it had the protection of a patent to cause the pharmaceutical company marketing it to promote its sale enthusiastically. Because it does not correct the underlying hormone disorder but instead stimulates ovulation in a relatively artificial manner, a smaller percentage of patients conceive with clomiphene therapy than with small doses of cortisone acetate or hydrocortisone, and of those who do conceive, a higher incidence of multiple births and of miscarriages occurs.[15, 16]

Patients treated with physiologic dosages of cortisone acetate or hydrocortisone, on the other hand, not only conceived, but they carried their pregnancies with an incidence of miscarriages no greater than that of the general population, provided the steroid was continued through the pregnancy.[14] In other words, small dosages of cortisone acetate or hydrocortisone seemed to protect against miscarriage as well as improve conception rate. For these reasons, small doses of cortisone acetate or hydrocortisone are preferable to clomiphene, and we have tried the latter only in patients who fail to respond to physiologic cortisone therapy. An occasional patient has conceived with clomiphene administration after low dosage glucocorticoid had failed, but numerous women have conceived on low dosage glucocorticoid therapy after having failed to conceive with clomiphene that had been prescribed prior to referral to me.

Most women who have androgenic changes such as acne and hirsutism associated with ovarian dysfunction have an increased excretion of urinary 17-KS or elevated levels of testosterone or DHA-sulfate in the blood, and the adequacy of treatment is reflected by the return of such measurements to normal. Hence, initially it was postulated that the ovarian dysfunction was caused by an excess of androgen. Later when it was found that dysfunction could occur without any excess androgen and still be corrected by small doses of cortisone acetate or hydrocortisone, it was concluded that an excessive production of estrogen by the adrenals, or at least under ACTH control, must be the cause of the disorder.[17, 18] An excessive production of estrogen can often be demonstrated in functional uterine bleeding, and the restoration of normal ovulatory cycles by small doses of glucocorticoids suggests that the excessive estrogen either was being produced by the adrenals or was under ACTH control. Precise determination of the extraovarian source of estrogen in patients with ovarian dysfunction has still not been achieved, however.

Two recent reports may be pertinent relative to the etiology of this type of hormonal disorder. Herrenkohl[19] has noted that prenatal stress of mother rats resulted in reduced fertility in their female offspring, with fewer conceptions, more spontaneous abortions and vaginal hemorrhages, longer pregnancies, lower birth weight, and fewer newborns likely to survive the neonatal period. Gupta et al.[20] reported that phenobarbital administration to pregnant rats also produced detrimental effects on reproductive function in their offspring, including delays in the onset of puberty, disorders in the estrous cycle, and infertility, associated with altered concentrations of sex steroids, gonadotrophic hormones, and estrogen receptors.

Other recent studies have brought to light another type of abnormality that can cause clinical disorders that might improve with physiologic dosages of glucocorticoid, namely, autoim-

mune phenomena. Because ovarian hormones as well as adrenocortical hormones are steroids, they do not stimulate the production of antibodies, but steroid hormone receptors are protein
molecules and, hence, can stimulate antibodies that could interfere with normal estrogen effect. Such cases might have normal
or elevated plasma estrogen levels, normal or slightly high plasma FSH, and amenorrhea or irregular menses. Breast development might also be poor. Ovarian dysfunction associated with
severe insulin resistance has been described as the "Type A
Syndrome,"[21] so it seems likely that ovarian dysfunction could
occur as an autoimmune disorder without insulin resistance. If
such occurs, the beneficial effect of glucocorticoids in autoimmune disorders, even in subreplacement dosages (Chapters 6, 7,
& 8), might account for favorable therapeutic responses.

Once the disturbed ovarian function has been corrected, the
remission may be maintained in some cases after the glucocorticoid has been discontinued, but most women seem to need to
continue the treatment indefinitely to maintain normal ovarian
function. We have not been able to follow a sufficient number of
daughters of patients with ovarian dysfunction into adolescence
to determine whether they can inherit this type of disorder, but
there is considerable evidence from patient histories that this
clinical problem does tend to be inherited.

It should be remembered that amenorrhea may be caused by
other disorders such as hypopituitarism, prolactin-producing
tumors of the pituitary, hypothyroidism, and primary ovarian
deficiency, as well as by congenital defects in genital development, and that irregular menses can result from relative ovarian
deficiency, but the majority of women with irregular menses,
secondary amenorrhea, functional uterine bleeding, and luteal
phase disorders will benefit from low dosage glucocorticoid
therapy, and associated infertility, if present, will often be
corrected.[14]

In the field of ovarian dysfunction some confusion has arisen
in the use of the term Stein-Leventhal syndrome. This syndrome
as originally described[22] included not only ovarian dysfunction
and androgenic changes but also bilateral polycystic enlargement of the ovaries. It has been found to be associated with an

abnormality of steroid metabolism in the ovaries, but in our experience, such patients usually require small doses of cortisone acetate or hydrocortisone in addition to small doses of estrogen to have a restoration of normal menstrual cycles and fertility. This syndrome, therefore, results from a more severe degree of steroid abnormality than is encountered in the majority of women with ovarian dysfunction and androgenic changes, so it does not seem wise to apply the term Stein-Leventhal syndrome to the milder, more common disorder. The tendency to apply the term loosely to all types of ovarian dysfunction is, therefore, misleading, and the diagnosis should be limited to those women who have not only ovarian dysfunction but also bilaterally enlarged polycystic ovaries. When the pathologic physiology of these disorders is more clearly characterized, it should be possible to differentiate them more precisely.

Several case histories demonstrate the promising potential and safety of low dosage glucocorticoid therapy in ovarian dysfunction.

Case 1

The patient was a seventeen year old female referred for primary amenorrhea. She had experienced slight breast development for several years but no spontaneous menses. Premarin, 1.25 mg daily for three weeks, plus Provera, 10 mg daily for the last five days, cyclically, for four months, had produced withdrawal flow but no subsequent menses. Her general health and energy had been good. She had no acne or hirsutism, and temperature tolerance was normal. She had no history of serious illness and no allergies. Her younger sister, age fifteen, had the menarche at age fourteen, and her cycles were regular but with a prolonged flow of nine days. The patient's paternal aunt had had a goiter removed, and grandparents on both sides had senile type of diabetes mellitus.

Physical examination revealed a pleasant, attractive girl with a clear complexion. Height was 67½ inches, weight 119½ pounds, blood pressure 90/60, pulse 76 and regular. She shaved her thighs but otherwise had no excessive hair growth. The thyroid was at the upper limits of normal in size, with no lymphadenopathy. Breast development was poor, and there were no masses. The remainder of the examination was normal except for slightly hypoactive reflexes. T_3 sponge uptake was 36 percent, and T_4 was 7.3 mcg%. Plasma estrogen was 185 pg/ml (normal 45-200), and plasma FSH 11.7 mIU/ml (normal 15-30). Plasma cortisol at 11:30 AM was 11.3 mcg%, a somewhat low value for that time of day; 30 minutes after an I.M. injection of 25 units of Cortrosyn, this rose to

27.7 mcg%, consistent with normal adrenal responsiveness.

The occurrence of high normal plasma estrogen and low plasma FSH in association with amenorrhea and subnormal breast development suggested either the production of abnormal estrogen, possibly under adrenal control, interfering with normal ovarian function, or some abnormality of estrogen receptors, possibly autoimmune in nature. Hydrocortisone (Cortef®), 5 mg four times daily, was therefore started. She returned six weeks later reporting considerable improvement in energy and sense of well-being, and she commented on having had no respiratory infections or influenza although two brothers and her father developed flu during an epidemic that was in progress at that time. There had also been much influenza at her school.

No evidence of ovulation occurred on basal temperature charts, however, and no menses occurred, so after three months, the dosage of hydrocortisone was increased to 7.5 mg four times daily. Within two weeks she had her first spontaneous menses. A month later T_3 sponge uptake was 51 percent, T_4 was 8.4 mcg%, and plasma estrogen was 49 pg/ml.

Although estrogen levels fluctuate during normal menstrual cycles, the decrease in plasma estrogen while the patient was taking hydrocortisone and after she had spontaneous menses suggested that the hydrocortisone had corrected either an excessive production of estrogen from some extra-ovarian source or an abnormality of estrogen receptors.

Because the patient's thyroid was still at the upper limit of normal in size, Euthroid, gr. ½ twice daily was added to her therapy. Subsequently basal temperature charts showed evidence of more regular ovulatory menstrual cycles, and breast development increased to normal. A repeat plasma estrogen determination was 73 pg/ml.

This case is an example of primary amenorrhea associated with a normal level of plasma estrogen and a low level of FSH. The poor breast development and lack of menses suggested that the estrogen was either not a normal type or that its physiologic effects were being blocked, and the relatively low baseline plasma cortisol suggested some adrenal disorder. She also had a slight nontoxic thyroid enlargement with a family history of goiter and diabetes mellitus, and her ovarian function did not show optimum improvement until suitable doses of thyroid medication were administered with the hydrocortisone. At the time she was studied, measurement of T_3 by RIA was not available, but recently a similar case has been encountered whose T_3 by RIA was low while T_3 sponge uptake and T_4 were normal.

This patient also appeared to have a high resistance to common respiratory illness and influenza while taking physiologic dosages of hydrocortisone in contrast to the resistance-impairing effects of large, pharmacologic dosages.

The patient in case 2 was also referred at the age of seventeen years, but she had secondary amenorrhea of eight months duration.

Case 2

The menarche had occurred at age ten, and cycles had been regular with intervals of twenty-eight to thirty days, menses lasting four days, until about eighteen months previously, when intervals increased up to two months and duration of flow decreased to two days. Menses stopped altogether eight months prior to the patient's referral. She had experienced acne since the menarche, treated since the previous summer with tetracycline, one tablet twice daily. She had also been receiving injections for allergic rhinitis and sinusitis for several years.

These injections had been discontinued at about the time of her last menstrual period, and her allergy symptoms had been worse in the spring before her visit. Thyroid enlargement had been noted intermittently since the previous summer. She had one sister, age sixteen, with regular cycles. Her maternal grandfather had diabetes and her father and paternal grandmother had hypertension. Physical examination revealed moderate acne of the face and slightly increased hair growth on her trunk. The thyroid was not enlarged. Breast development was normal with no masses. Blood pressure was 100/75, pulse 92 and regular. Height was 64 ¾ inches, weight 117 pounds. Pelvic examination was normal, with no enlargement of the ovaries. Urinary 17-KS were 13.9 and 17-OHST 3.9 mg/24 hours.

The patient was given hydrocortisone, 2.5 mg four times daily, and she returned two months later reporting that a spontaneous menstrual period lasting four days had occurred. She also reported significant improvement in her complexion, although she had discontinued tetracycline several weeks previously. Allergic symptoms had also improved. She was reluctant to continue to take the hydrocortisone, however, because she had read reports of the hazardous potential of glucocorticoid therapy, and after she had been getting along well for several months, she discontinued it. Her cycles continued to be fairly regular, but she experienced exacerbation of her acne and allergies after the hydrocortisone was stopped.

Conjugated estrogen (Premarin), 0.3 mg daily except during menses, was then tried. This produced impressive improvement in her acne, but her allergies seemed worse, so hydrocortisone, 5 mg four times daily, was resumed. On this program she did quite well, with regular menstrual cycles, few allergic symptoms, and only occasional mild acne. Several years later when she read news reports regarding the possible harmful effects of Premarin, she discontinued it. Her cycles continued regular on the hydrocortisone, and her complexion remained clear.

This patient is an example of a young woman with secondary amenorrhea and acne that responded to small doses of hydrocortisone. Her acne also improved with a small dosage of Premarin, but this did not help her allergic symptoms, whereas hydrocortisone had benefited her acne, her allergic symptoms, and her ovarian dysfunction. Her case also demonstrates how some patients with acne who have been treated with tetracycline can discontinue the tetracycline when they receive suitable dosages of hydrocortisone. Her experience further emphasizes the need for the news media to report the value of safe dosages as well as the potential harm of excessive dosages of normal hormones. The tendency for the news media to dramatize the hazardous aspects of therapy with adrenocortical and ovarian hormones without pointing out the safety and need for physiologic dosages of these hormones in patients with certain types of hormone deficiency has become a serious problem.

Case 3 is an example of a type of ovarian dysfunction seen somewhat more frequently in recent years.

Case 3

This woman was referred at the age of twenty-two years because of secondary amenorrhea. The menarche had occurred at age twelve, with fairly regular cycles for approximately two years, but they then became irregular with intervals of twenty-one to sixty days, menses lasting five days with severe cramps. At age eighteen she was given an oral contraceptive to regulate her cycles, and she also married during that year. The oral contraceptive was discontinued three years later, but she had no subsequent spontaneous menses. She had experienced increased hair growth since age thirteen or fourteen, but this had apparently diminished while she was taking the oral contraceptive. Two lumps had been noted in the right breast, and they had subsided after aspiration.

Physical examination revealed a height of 65½ inches, weight 152 pounds, blood pressure 90/70, pulse 88 and regular. There was moderately excessive hair growth on the face, trunk, and extremities. The thyroid was not enlarged. Breast development was normal with no masses. The clitoris was not enlarged. The remainder of her examination was not remarkable. Urinary 17-KS were 31.5 mg/24 hours. Blood

FSH was 5.2 mIU/ml, total estrogens 19.6 pg/ml, and plasma testosterone was less than 30 ng/dl. Plasma cortisol at 11 AM was 9.3 mcg%; thirty minutes after an I.M. injection of 25 units of Cortrosyn, this rose to 42.3 mcg%. Urinary 17-KS after dexamethasone suppression decreased to 9.2 mg/24 hours.

On hydrocortisone, 5 mg four times daily, urinary 17-KS decreased to 17.6 mg/24 hours, so the dosage was increased to 7.5 mg four times daily. She was also given a 1200 calorie diet on which she lost 17 pounds. On this program she resumed having regular ovulatory cycles, and urinary 17-KS were 13 mg/24 hours. She did not wish to become pregnant. In early 1976 she reported that her cycles were regular and that she had been the only one in her entire department at work who had not had influenza during that spring epidemic. Twelve others were quite sick and missed many days from work.

This type of disorder, in which ovarian function is apparently normal for several years, progressing to irregular menses and associated with androgenic changes, often progresses to amenorrhea spontaneously, but in this case the administration of an oral contraceptive for several years preceded the amenorrhea. The apparent aggravation of ovarian dysfunction after a prolonged course of an oral contraceptive has been observed in other patients and suggests that it may be advisable for patients with ovarian dysfunction to avoid use of oral contraceptives. The elevated urinary 17-KS excretion with normal plasma testosterone levels was consistent with the production of an excess of androgen other than testosterone. The responses to dexamethasone and to hydrocortisone also indicate that the excess androgen was under ACTH control. The improvement in hair growth that apparently occurred while she was taking the oral contraceptive has been observed in other patients and suggests that the oral contraceptive can affect adrenocortical function as well as ovarian function. Finally, the failure of this patient to develop influenza during an epidemic that affected everyone else in her department at work was impressive and indicated that this therapy certainly was not impairing her resistance to infection.

Case number 4 is an example of the beneficial effect of cortisone or hydrocortisone therapy in a patient with functional uterine bleeding.

Case 4

This sixteen year old girl was referred because of irregular menses and prolonged bleeding. The menarche had occurred at age fourteen, and cycles had always been irregular with intervals of two to six months, menses lasting eight days with occasional cramps. She had noted acne for about a year and also some increase in hair growth on her abdomen. For the previous six weeks she had been spotting continuously. Her general health was good. She had a history of an appendectomy for a ruptured appendix at age nine, and there was a family history of goiter on both maternal and paternal sides.

Physical examination revealed an attractive young woman with mild increased hair growth in the periareolar and subumbilical areas. The thyroid was not enlarged; blood pressure was 90/60, pulse 72 and regular, height was 63 inches, weight 102½ pounds. Neither the clitoris nor the ovaries was enlarged. Urinary 17-KS were 13.5 mg/24 hours. She was given progesterone, 5 mg by mouth daily for five days to produce an initial withdrawal flow, and Cortef, 5 mg four times daily. On this medication she resumed regular ovulatory cycles, but she continued to complain of sensitivity to cold, and her energy did not return completely to normal. In August, 1972, T_3 sponge uptake was 65 percent and T_4 was 4.0 mcg%. She was given a prescription for Euthroid, gr. 1½ daily with impressive improvement in energy and less sensitivity to cold.

A year later, when she went to college, she discontinued the Euthroid and took the Cortef irregularly. If her menstrual period was late, she would take the Cortef until it developed. In January of her freshman year she had infectious mononucleosis, but she did not increase the dosage of Cortef. She stopped Cortef altogether in the spring of her sophomore year and during the subsequent year she developed progressive dysmenorrhea, with nausea and vomiting at the onset of her menses. When she returned for follow-up in the spring of her junior year, plasma cortisol at 2:15 PM was 11.6 μg%; thirty minutes after an I.M. injection of 25 units of Cortrosyn, plasma cortisol rose to 31.2 μg%. Plasma FSH was 6.0 and plasma estrogen was 125 pg/ml. T_3 sponge uptake was 63 percent, and T_4 was 6.9 mcg%. She was instructed to resume Cortef, 5 mg four times daily, and Euthroid, gr. 1 daily, and she had a resumption of normal cycles and improvement in energy.

Features worthy of comment in this case include irregular menses from the menarche and flow lasting eight days. The occurrence of relatively prolonged flow with regular cycles may be a manifestation of mild hypothyroidism, but irregularity of the cycles is more frequently associated with a disorder of steroid metabolism. The development of metropathia is usually associated with an excessive production of estrogen, either from the adrenals or under ACTH control, that interferes with normal ovarian function and is corrected by physiologic dosages of cortisone acetate or hydrocortisone. The history of a ruptured appendix at age nine is interesting because a number of other patients with ovarian dysfunction have given histories of having had a severe illness in childhood, suggesting that severe stress may predispose to this type of endocrine disorder. Administration of Provera is helpful in patients with metropathia to produce withdrawal flow because the pathologic physiology is an excessive stimulation of the endometrium by persistent estrogen production without the cyclic shedding that follows ovulation. The "medical D. & C." produced by Provera therefore prevents persistent bleeding during the interval before the effects of corrective hormone therapy occur. A dosage of 5 mg Provera daily for five days seems to be preferable to 10 mg on the same schedule because it produces withdrawal flow yet is not as apt to inhibit ovulation as the larger dosage. It is not unusual for the 5 mg dose to stimulate an ovulation, in which case menstruation does not occur until approximately fourteen days later, instead of the two to four day interval that occurs without ovulation.

Girls with metropathia frequently have mild hypothyroidism, and the response to Euthroid in this case was impressive, although T_3 sponge uptake and T_4 were within low normal range. The measurement of T_3 by RIA provides a means of detecting a decreased ability to convert T_4 to T_3 as a possible cause of thyroid deficiency in such cases at present, but this test was not available at the time this patient was studied. Of additional interest in this case is that ovarian dysfunction did not remain corrected after she discontinued medication, but it returned in somewhat milder form and persisted until Cortef and Euthroid were resumed.

Case 5 is an example of a girl with functional uterine bleeding that eventually progressed to amenorrhea.

Case 5

The patient was referred at age sixteen with a history of irregular prolonged uterine bleeding since the menarche at age twelve. Intervals between menses had been as long as six months and duration of flow as long as three weeks. A dilatation and curettage had been performed at age twelve, and subsequently she had been given an oral contraceptive for several months without benefit. Her last menstrual period had occurred ten months previously. Plasma FSH was 9.2 mIU/ml (normal 6-30), plasma total estrogens were 56 pg/ml (normal for preovulatory phase was 100-200; this was run by a different laboratory from that used for previous cases), T_3 sponge uptake was 53 percent, and T_4 was 6.7 mcg%, both well within normal limits. Plasma cortisol at 1:30 PM was 14.0; one hour after an I.M. injection of 25 units of ACTH, this rose to 37.3 mcg%.

She was given Cortef, 5 mg four times daily, and plasma estrogens increased to 175 pg/ml, but she failed to ovulate. Synthroid, 0.1 mg daily, was added, later increasing to 0.15 mg daily, but she did not ovulate until the dosage was increased to 0.2 mg daily. She is now having regular ovulatory cycles on Cortef, 5 mg four times daily, plus Synthroid, 0.2 mg daily.

This girl had metropathia from the menarche at age twelve. Such patients are often given an oral contraceptive in a cyclic fashion to produce regular withdrawal flow, but this type of therapy does not usually help the fundamental disorder, and in some cases it seems to aggravate it. Prior to the availability of oral contraceptives these patients were sometimes treated with cyclic estrogen and progesterone in physiologic dosages, and this therapy occasionally seemed to stimulate ovulatory cycles after it was withdrawn, but patients frequently relapsed to metropathia within a few months. In this case the normal plasma FSH with low total estrogens suggested the presence of estrogens that were not being measured in the assay. Hydrocortisone therapy resulted in an increase in plasma estrogen level, consistent with an abnormality in steroid metabolism, but ovulation did not occur until she also received thyroid in a sufficient dosage, even though T_3 sponge uptake and T_4 had been normal prior to therapy. Patients with metropathia frequently require physiologic dosages of thyroid medication as well as hydrocortisone or cortisone acetate, suggesting an associated mild thyroid deficiency even though T_3 sponge uptake and T_4 may be within normal limits. As stated previously, T_3 by RIA is a more sensitive indicator of thyroid function, but this test was not available at the time this patient was studied.

Case 6 is an example of ovarian and thyroid dysfunction with infertility.

Case 6

This twenty-five year old female was referred because of a thyroid disorder, irregular menses, and infertility. The menarche had occurred at age eleven, and cycles had always been irregular with intervals of four to six weeks, menses lasting three to five days with cramps. She had experienced acne since the menarche, and hirsutism for the previous two years. She was married at age twenty, took an oral contraceptive from age twenty to age twenty-three, and had used no precautions for eighteen months prior to her visit. After stopping the oral contraceptive, she developed abdominal pain and had a laparatomy for a "pseudocyst" of the ovary. When she failed to conceive, she received a bilateral wedge resection for sclerocystic ovaries six months prior to her referral. Meanwhile she had been given injections of a progestational agent to try to correct her ovarian function. After the wedge resection she had two menses a month apart, then cycles became irregular again. Her energy had been poor for about five years, she was sensitive to cold and had a tendency to constipation. She had experienced frequent palpitations and tremor in the previous year. Her brother was married and had two children. Her mother had ovarian dysfunction and had had difficulty in conceiving.

Physical examination revealed a height of 67 inches, weight 137½ pounds, blood pressure 124/80, pulse 96 and regular. There was mild acne of the chin and mild periareolar hair. The thyroid was two-and-one-half times normal size, rather firm, with no lymphadenopathy. Breasts were hypoplastic, but within lower limits of normal and contained no masses. Heart, lungs, and abdomen were normal except for laparatomy scars. Reflexes were equal and hyperactive. T_3 sponge uptake was 52 percent. T_4 was 6.2 mcg%, thyroid antibodies were negative, total estrogen was 47 pg/ml (normal 100-200), plasma cortisol at 4 PM was 14.0, and thirty minutes after an I.M. injection of 25 units of Cortrosyn this rose to 39.3 mcg%.

She was given Euthroid, gr. 1 daily, and Cortef, 5 mg four times daily. A month later her thyroid had returned to normal size and her menstrual cycles became more regular with evidence of ovulation on the twelfth to fourteenth days of twenty-five to twenty-eight day cycles, but she failed to conceive.

Plasma estrogen was 133 pg/ml. Premarin, 0.3 mg daily except during menses, was added to her regimen and she conceived in the second cycle after this program was started. After conception, T_3 sponge uptake was 38 percent, and T_4 was 8.1 mcg%, but her thyroid began to enlarge, so the dosage of Euthroid was increased to gr. 1 twice a day, Cortef being continued at 5 mg four times daily. She had a full term, normal delivery and nursed her baby for a month.

Because her tubes reportedly showed considerable scarring, her obstetrician advised another pregnancy as soon as possible. After delivery she resumed Cortef, 5 mg four times daily, and Euthroid, gr. 1 daily. The Premarin had been discontinued as soon as her pregnancy had been diagnosed, and this was not resumed. She had two normal cycles and then conceived again. Euthroid was again increased to gr. 1 twice daily, the Cortef continued at 5 mg four times daily, and she delivered a normal female infant by breech three weeks early. She did not nurse this baby, and menses resumed normally.

This patient was an example of the Stein-Leventhal syndrome with only transient improvement following wedge resection. She also had a nontoxic goiter with a normal T_3 sponge uptake and T_4. Plasma estrogen was low, but plasma FSH was in the low normal range, suggesting that she was either producing an estrogen that was not being measured or that pituitary function was mildly impaired. On a combination of Euthroid and Cortef she resumed regular menstrual cycles, and her thyroid returned to normal size, but she failed to conceive until a small dose of estrogen was added. She had a second pregnancy on Cortef and Euthroid but without the estrogen. This case typifies the necessity of having not only ovarian but also adrenal and thyroid function normal before conception can occur.

In our earlier experience with this type of therapy we suggested that after delivery women continue the physiologic dosage of glucocorticoid until they had resumed regular ovulatory cycles and then try stopping so as to determine whether they would maintain normal ovarian function.[1] On the basis of subsequent experience it appears that most patients remain more normal if they continue to take the small doses of glucocorticoid indefinitely.

Case number 7 is that of a seventeen year old girl with metropathia associated with elevated plasma estrogen apparently related to emotional stress.

Case 7

The patient had the menarche at age eleven, and her cycles were regular with intervals of twenty-eight days, menses lasting four to five days. At age fifteen she developed emotional problems, for which she was treated with Thorazine®. She then began to have frequent, prolonged menses with intervals of two to three weeks, flow lasting up to three weeks. She had been given an oral contraceptive for three months without benefit. She tended to tire easily and for several years had been sensitive to both heat and cold. She had mild premenstrual acne and in recent months had also noted increased hair growth on her upper lip. During the previous year she had frequent sore throats, and a tonsillectomy had been recommended. During this year her weight increased from 115 pounds to 154 pounds in spite of attempts to diet. In the previous two weeks she had experienced frequent headaches. She drank four large glasses of cola daily and had been smoking one and a half packs of cigarettes daily for five years. One of her three sisters had metropathia, and her mother was reported to have high blood pressure.

Physical examination revealed a stocky female with mild acne of the chin and mild increased hair growth on her upper lip and trunk. Height was 63 inches, weight 154¼ pounds, blood pressure 120/70, pulse 92 and regular. The thyroid was not enlarged. Breast development was normal, with no masses. The remainder of her examination was not remarkable. T_3 sponge uptake was 40 percent, T_4 was 8.0 mcg%, and plasma FSH was 11.7 mIU/ml, all normal values. Plasma estrogen was 356 (normal 45-200) and plasma estradiol 282 pg/ml (normal 15-75). Plasma cortisol at 9 AM was 21.1, and thirty minutes after an I.M. injection of 25 units of Cortrosyn this rose to 33.1 mcg%.

These findings were consistent with low adrenal reserve with an excessive production of total estrogen and estradiol. Plasma FSH was normal, rather than low, as would be expected with elevated estrogen. She was given Provera, 5 mg daily for five days, to produce withdrawal flow, and Cortef, 5 mg four times daily, to correct the steroid disorder. She was also given instructions for a 1200 calorie reduction diet and to decrease her intake of caffeine and use of tobacco. She failed to lose weight, but on this program she resumed regular ovulatory cycles with intervals of twenty-six, twenty-seven, twenty-eight, and twenty-three days, respectively, the latter cycle being complicated by a strep throat. Plasma total estrogen and estradiol levels returned to normal, although she continued to take psychotropic medication.

The development of ovarian dysfunction at the time she had emotional problems is consistent with the known tendency for stress to cause ovarian dysfunction in women who have a predisposition to such disorders, but psychotropic drugs can also cause ovarian dysfunction, so the taking of Thorazine may have contributed to this disorder.

Case 8 is that of a twenty-four year old female who was born and raised in Europe, moved to the United States at age sixteen, was married at age twenty-one, had used no precautions and had no pregnancies.

Case 8

The menarche had occurred at age thirteen, and cycles had been regular with intervals of twenty-seven to twenty-nine days, menses lasting four days without cramps. She had no acne. Frequency of intercourse was adequate. General health and energy had been good. Her hands and feet would get cold easily. She had no allergies. Her mother had some difficulty conceiving but eventually had two full-term, normal deliveries. Her husband had fathered a child by a previous marriage. Family history was negative for endocrine disorder.

Physical examination revealed a rather tall, well-developed, well-nourished young woman with no acne. The thyroid was soft, at upper limits of normal in size. Breasts were clear. There were a few periareolar and subumbilical hairs. Heart, lungs, and abdomen were normal. There was no edema. T_3 sponge uptake was 39.5 percent, and T_4 was 9.8 μg%, both normal values. Urinary 17-KS were 17.5 mg/24 hours and 17-OHST 16.4 mg/24 hours. Plasma cortisol at 8 AM was 21.2 μg%; one hour after an I.M. injection of ACTH, this rose to 34.5 μg%, consistent with low adrenal reserve.

Because of the suggestive slight thyroid enlargement, she was initially given Euthroid, gr. 1 daily for four months. During this time basal temperature charts showed ovulations in cycles lasting twenty-seven to thirty-six days with good exposure but no conception. Cortef, 5 mg four times daily, was then added. Basal temperature charts showed evidence of ovulation nine days after Cortef had been begun, and she conceived with that ovulation. Cortef and Euthroid were continued in the same dosage up to the time of delivery of an 8 pound, 15 ounce, full-term, normal male infant.

This case is an example of how a history of regular menses does not rule out a mild hormone disorder as a cause of infertility. The presence of a small, nontoxic goiter indicated the need for thyroid medication, but conception did not occur until hydrocortisone was added.

REPEATED MISCARRIAGES

As noted previously, women who have difficulty conceiving also have a high incidence of miscarriages, but when the physiologic dosages of glucocorticoid that are administered to correct the mild disorder of steroid metabolism or possible autoimmune disorder that interferes with their conceiving are continued throughout the pregnancy, the incidence of miscarriages is not greater than that of women who have no difficulty conceiving. In other words, continuation of the physiologic dosages of cortisone or hydrocortisone during a pregnancy helps to protect against miscarriage in this type of disorder.

For women who have repeated miscarriages without any apparent abnormality of their menstrual cycles, the administration of suitable doses of thyroid medication sufficient to bring the plasma thyroxine level above 8.0 mcg% is often beneficial in protecting the pregnancy.[18, 23] Some women require both small dosages of cortisone acetate or hydrocortisone and supplementary thyroid medication to prevent miscarriages.

Women who have difficulty conceiving should therefore have plasma thyroxine levels checked after conception, and if they do not rise above 8 mcg% within a month, the administration of sufficient thyroid medication to bring the level above 8 mcg% may help to protect against miscarriage. Because an occasional patient becomes resistant to extracts of animal thyroid glands, I prefer to prescribe synthetic preparations of sodium-L-thyroxine or sodium-L-thyroxine plus triiodothyronine. Daily dosages equivalent to one or two grains of additional thyroid medication daily are sufficient in most cases.

A woman who has corrected her difficulty in conceiving by taking small doses of hydrocortisone or cortisone acetate should continue this medication through pregnancy up to the time of delivery. These small, physiologic dosages do not harm the mother or her baby, and they seem to be necessary, in at least some cases, to enable the mother to maintain a normal pregnancy. Because they do not impair resistance to stress, there is no need to administer additional glucocorticoid at the time of delivery, even if Caesarean section is necessary, unless the mother had previous evidence of adrenal insufficiency or low adrenal reserve. If she had such evidence, the administration of 50 mg Solu-Cortef intramuscularly every eight hours during labor or 100 mg intramuscularly one hour prior to Caesarean section, followed by 50 mg every eight hours for twenty-four hours, then 25 mg intramuscularly every eight hours until oral medication can be resumed seems to protect against relative adrenal insufficiency without causing any harm to either the mother or her baby. After spontaneous vaginal delivery, the steroid can be resumed in the same maintenance dosage that had been taken during pregnancy as soon as the mother is able to take oral medication, and it may be continued through nursing without harm to the mother or her baby.

When thyroid medication is given to protect against miscarriage, it should be continued up to delivery, but after delivery the dosage of thyroid should be reduced to the prepregnancy level. A woman not only needs but is also more tolerant of larger dosages of thyroid during a pregnancy, but if these larger dosages are continued into the postpartum period, symptoms of hyperthyroidism may develop.

The pathologic physiology of repeated miscarriages is not fully understood. After a woman becomes pregnant, her T_3 sponge uptake normally decreases and serum T_4 increases, reflecting the increase in thyroxine-binding globulin that occurs with increased estrogen activity, and patients with repeated miscarriages frequently fail to show these changes. One could postulate that the problem results from an inadequate production of estrogen, but the administration of estrogen to such patients does not seem to help to protect the pregnancy, and there are reports that some types of estrogen administration during pregnancy may be harmful. These seem to apply primarily to artificial estrogens such as diethylstilbestrol, but until this question is clarified, it is considered inadvisable to administer estrogen during pregnancy.

Evidence that placental synthesis of estrogen is closely linked to the supply of circulating dehydroepiandrosterone sulfate and hence to adrenocortical activity may be pertinent,[24] but the effect of cortisone or thyroid hormone administration upon DHA sulfate levels in women with repeated miscarriages has not been reported.

An excessive production of prostaglandins can cause miscarriage, but I have not seen any report that women with repeated miscarriages produce excessive amounts of prostaglandins, nor have I seen any report that administration of thyroid hormone or glucocorticoids affects prostaglandin production. It is possible that the protection against hypoglycemia provided by glucocorticoids may contribute to their protective effect. It is also possible that an abnormality of estrogen receptor function may be at fault.

One might be concerned that protection of pregnancies under such circumstances might cause patients to carry abnormal fetuses to term, but in our experience this has not occurred. We have been able to obtain information on a total of 209 babies that have been borne by women who have taken physiologic dosages of cortisone acetate or hydrocortisone throughout their pregnancies. These have included ninety boys, ninety-five girls, and twenty-four babies whose sex was not reported to us. Caesarean section was performed in twenty-seven instances on twenty-one patients, twice with each of three mothers and three times with one mother. Two sets of twins occurred. Only six of these 209 babies were reported to have congenital abnormalities; three had mild defects that were only temporary or easily corrected, whereas three had more serious disorders, including one Down's syndrome, one dislocated hip, and one infant with multiple congenital defects that died six hours after birth. This was the only fatality in the 209 infants. This incidence of congenital defects in six of 209 babies is 2.9 percent, the same as the incidence of congenital malformations in live births in the general population.

Case 9 is an example of a woman with repeated miscarriages and no other apparent evidence of endocrine disorder who was helped by cortisone therapy.

Case 9

This young woman was referred to me in 1959, at age twenty-five, because of repeated miscarriages. She had reached the menarche at age sixteen, and cycles were regular at thirty day intervals, menses lasted five days without cramps. She had been married two years previously. During her first pregnancy she started spotting in her sixth week, was given some injections and some tablets (she could not identify these) but had a D. & C. for missed abortion in her fourth month. In her second pregnancy she again started spotting at her sixth week, was given some tablets but miscarried at eight weeks. In her third pregnancy she started spotting and miscarried at six weeks gestation. During this pregnancy she took no medication. Her energy was poor, and she was sensitive to cold. Most women notice an increased sensation of warmth and sensitivity to heat during a normal pregnancy, but she had noted no change in temperature tolerance during her pregnancies. Her mother had difficulty becoming pregnant, finally conceiving the patient after eight years, and she had no subsequent pregnancies. Her father had diabetes mellitus of recent onset.

Physical examination was within normal limits with no enlargement of the thyroid gland. PBI was 5.8 mcg%, and I^{131} uptake was 31 percent in twenty-four hours, both normal values. Response to TSH stimulation was normal. Urinary 17-KS were 10.4 mg/24 hrs, also normal. Her basal temperature chart showed evidence of ovulation on the fourteenth day of thirty day cycles. On sodium-L-thyroxine, 0.1 mg daily, her energy improved somewhat, and with the addition of cortisone acetate, 2.5 mg four times daily, her energy increased further. She then conceived again; a month after conception, PBI was 6.8 mcg%, so the dosage of Synthroid was increased to 0.2 mg daily. She had slight spotting just before the dosage was increased, but it subsided after she stayed off her feet for two days. A month later PBI was 10.3 mcg%, and she carried her pregnancy to term without further problems, having a Caesarean section. After delivery the cortisone was discontinued and thyroxine dosage decreased to 0.1 mg daily. She nursed her baby for six weeks, and menses resumed spontaneously three months post partum. She conceived again eight months after her first delivery, this time while taking only thyroxine, 0.1 mg daily. Her dosage was increased to 0.2 mg daily three weeks after conception. She began spotting at that time, and this continued for about two weeks, then stopped. At seven weeks gestation PBI was 7.6 mcg%. Spotting resumed in her eighth week, and she miscarried shortly thereafter.

Four months later menses had resumed normally, but there was evidence of chronic cystic mastitis. Cortisone acetate, 2.5 mg four times daily, was resumed in addition to the thyroxine, 0.1 mg daily, and the patient reported impressive improvement in her energy; examination revealed the cystic mastitis had cleared. She conceived again shortly afterwards. Thyroxine was increased to 0.2 mg daily and cortisone acetate continued at 2.5 mg four times daily throughout her pregnancy, which was normal, ending in a full-term Caesarean section. After delivery she resumed cortisone acetate, 2.5 mg four times daily, and continued thyroxine, 0.1 mg daily, because she said she felt much better while taking these medications.

An ACTH test performed six months after her second delivery revealed baseline urinary 17-KS of 7.5 mg/24 hours and cortisol metabolites of 10.1 mg/24 hours. After 80 units of ACTH gel intramuscularly, urinary 17-KS increased to 8.6 and cortisol metabolites to 32.3 mg/24 hours.

The patient did not desire further pregnancies, so she had a tubal ligation. Thyroid medication was discontinued at age thirty-seven without apparent symptomatic change. An ACTH test at age thirty-seven, while she was taking cortisone acetate, 2.5 mg four times daily, revealed a baseline plasma cortisol of 17.1 mcg% at 9 AM; one hour after an I.M. injection of 25 units of ACTH this rose to 40.6 mcg%, consistent with normal adrenal responsiveness. She was therefore advised to try stopping the cortisone acetate, and four months later a repeat ACTH test revealed a baseline plasma cortisol at 9:15 AM of 30.5 mcg%; one hour after an I.M. injection of 25 units of ACTH this rose to 71.2 mcg%. She has continued to feel well for the subsequent seven years.

This case demonstrated several interesting points. After having had three miscarriages in the first trimester, the patient had a full-term normal pregnancy on a combination of sodium-L-thyroxine and cortisone acetate, the latter in a dosage of only 2.5 mg four times daily. Subsequently, on thyroxine alone, she miscarried again. It is interesting to note that her serum PBI was 10.3 mcg% while taking thyroxine, 0.2 mg daily, during the pregnancy that she carried to term, and that it was only 7.6 mcg% while taking the same dosage of thyroxine during the pregnancy that miscarried. This suggests that the small dosage of cortisone acetate had in some way helped to increase the PBI level during pregnancy. She subsequently had another full-term normal pregnancy when cortisone acetate was given with the thyroxine in the same dosage as in the first pregnancy.

After having taken these normal hormones in small dosages for over twenty years, they were discontinued without any return of chronic fatigue, which had been the only subjective symptom that had responded to the therapy. It is therefore evident that prolonged treatment did not cause the patient to become dependent upon these medications but rather seemed to help enable her to continue to feel better after she stopped them.

TESTICULAR DYSFUNCTION

It is logical to assume that if mild adrenal dysfunction can produce disorders of ovarian function in women, it can produce disorders of testicular function in men, because an excess of androgen or estrogen can impair normal spermatogenesis. Small doses of cortisone acetate or hydrocortisone have therefore been administered to men with oligospermia, and an impressive number (about 50 percent) have had a significant rise in sperm count with this therapy.[25] Because normal human spermatozoa require about two months to mature, treatment should be continued for at least three months to determine whether it is being helpful. Some men with oligospermia may have elevated urinary 17-KS excretion, but most have a normal or relatively low excretion of these steroids. Some have elevated levels of plasma estrogen that can be suppressed to normal with small doses of hydrocortisone, and some have mild gynecomastia. The dosages of cortisone acetate or hydrocortisone are similar to those used for ovarian dysfunction. A possible reason that men have a lower percentage of response to this type of therapy is my impression that they sometimes do not seem to have as great an incentive to follow a detailed therapeutic program for fertility as carefully as their wives do, and this type of therapy must be followed meticulously to be maximally effective.

REFERENCES

1. Jefferies WMcK, Weir WC, Weir DR, Prouty RL: The use of cortisone and related steroids in infertility. *Fertil Steril 9:*145-166, 1958.
2. Jefferies WMcK, Michelakis AM: Individual patterns of urinary 17-ketosteroid fractions. *Metabolism 12:*1017-1031, 1963.
3. Jefferies WMcK: Low dosage glucocorticoid therapy. *Arch Intern Med 119:*265-278, 1967.
4. Hench PS, Kendall EC, Slocumb CH, Polley HF: The effect of a hormone of the adrenal cortex (17-hydroxy-11-dehydrocorticosterone: Compound E) and of pituitary adrenocorticotropic hormone on rheumatoid arthritis. Preliminary report. *Proc Staff Meet Mayo Clin 24:*181-197, 1949.
5. Slocumb CH, Polley HF, Hench PS, Kendall EC: Effects of cortisone and ACTH on patients with rheumatoid arthritis. *Proc Staff Meet Mayo Clin 25:*476-478, 1950.
6. Andrews RV: Influence of adrenal gland on gonadal function. In Thomas JA, Singhal RL (Eds.): *Advances in Sex Hormone Research, Vol. 3: Regulatory Mechanisms Affecting Gonadal Hormone Action.* Baltimore, Univ Park, 1976, pp. 197-215.
7. Kitay JI: Pituitary-adrenal function in the rat after gonadectomy and gonadal hormone replacement. *Endocrinology 73:*253-260, 1964.
8. Kitay JI, Coyne MD, Newsome W, Nelson R: Relation of the ovary to adrenal corticosterone production and adrenal enzyme activity in the rat. *Endocrinology 77:*902-908, 1965.
9. Colby HD, Kitay JI: Effects of gonadal hormones on adrenocortical secretion of 5-reduced metabolites of corticosterone in the rat. *Endocrinology 91:*1523-1527, 1972.

10. Jefferies WMcK, Levy RP: Treatment of ovarian dysfunction with small doses of cortisone or hydrocortisone. *J Clin Endocrinol Metab 19:*1069-1080, 1959.

11. Jefferies WMcK: Further experience with small doses of cortisone and related steroids in infertility associated with ovarian dysfunction. *Fertil Steril 11:*100-108, 1960.

12. Jefferies WMcK: Effect of small doses of cortisone upon urinary 17-ketosteroid fractions in patients with ovarian dysfunction. *J Clin Endocrinol Metab 22:*255-260, 1962.

13. Jefferies WMcK: Effects of low-dosage steroid therapy on 17-ketosteroid fractions in infertility. *Fertil Steril 14:*342-351, 1963.

14. Jefferies WMcK: Glucocorticoids and ovulation. In Greenblatt RB (Ed.): *Ovulation.* Philadelphia, Lippincott, 1966, pp. 62-74.

15. Karow WG, Payne SA: Pregnancy after clomiphene citrate treatment. *Fertil Steril 19:*351-362, 1968.

16. Seegar Jones G, Maffezzoli RD, Strott CA, Ross GT, Kaplan G: Pathophysiology of reproductive failure after clomiphene-induced ovulation. *Am J Obstet Gynecol 108:*847-867, 1970.

17. Jefferies WMcK: Treatment of ovarian dysfunction with cortisone or estrogen. *J Miss State Med Assoc 8:*279-283, 1967.

18. Jefferies WMcK: Thyroid and adrenal problems in gynecology. In Caplan RM, Sweeney WJ III, (Eds.): *Advances in Obstetrics and Gynecology.* Baltimore, Williams & Wilkins, 1978, pp. 394-401.

19. Herrenkohl LR: Prenatal stress reduces fertility and fecundity in female offspring. *Science 206:*1097-1099, 1979.

20. Gupta C, Sonawane BR, Yaffe SJ, Shapiro BH: Phenobarbital exposure in utero: Alterations in female reproductive function in rats. *Science 208:*508-510, 1980.

21. Flier JS, Kahn CR, Roth J: Receptors, antireceptor antibodies and mechanisms of insulin resistance. *N Engl J Med 300:*413-419, 1979.

22. Stein IF: Bilateral polycystic ovaries; significance in sterility. *Am J Obstet Gynecol 50:*385-398, 1945.

23. Jefferies WMcK: Symposium on ovarian dysfunction: The endocrine glands other than the gonads. *Clin Obstet Gynecol 8:*73-90, 1965.

24. MacDonald PC, Siiteri PK: Origin of estrogen in women pregnant with anencephalic foetus. *J Clin Invest 44:*465-474, 1965.

25. Jefferies, WMcK: Hormonal therapy of male infertility. *Urol Dig 6:*13-16, 1967.

Chapter 6

PHYSIOLOGIC DOSAGES IN RHEUMATIC DISORDERS INCLUDING RHEUMATOID ARTHRITIS

THE ANTIARTHRITIC EFFECTS of large doses of glucocorticoids are well-known. As has been mentioned previously, arthritis was the first pathologic disorder other than adrenal insufficiency for which glucocorticoid therapy was administered clinically, and because of the type of preparation and schedule of administration, the early dosages were much larger than what was later found to be a physiologic replacement dosage. When undesirable and hazardous side effects were encountered with such large dosages, it was assumed that any dosage would be dangerous. There has, therefore, been a tendency to avoid glucocorticoid therapy in arthritic conditions except as a last resort and then to discontinue it as soon as possible.

The evidence that cortisone acetate and hydrocortisone can be administered in safe dosages that may be taken indefinitely without harmful side effects raised the question of whether such safe dosages might have a place in the treatment of rheumatoid arthritis. An interesting report of one of the early patients with rheumatoid arthritis treated with cortisone acetate[1] implies that after initial dosages of 50 mg intramuscularly twice daily he was satisfactorily maintained on oral dosages of 50 mg and later 35 mg per day. The schedule of administration was not mentioned. Unfortunately, he subsequently died of intestinal hemorrhage, possibly related to potassium chloride, ascorbic acid, and aspirin that were also taken, but the implication of antiarthritic effects of smaller dosages of cortisone was clear.

Twelve years ago I reported the beneficial effects of *physiologic* dosages of cortisone acetate or hydrocortisone on two patients with rheumatoid arthritis, with evidence that patients with rheumatoid arthritis seemed to have a lower excretion of dehydroepiandrosterone in their urine and, hence, might have a mild

93

abnormality of steroid metabolism.[2] Hill and Dempsey[3] had reported a similar abnormality in steroid excretion pattern in rheumatoid arthritis several years previously.

A review of the literature fails to reveal any attempts by others to confirm these observations or even any comment on them. The benefit of low dosage glucocorticoid therapy in menopausal arthritis is exemplified in Case 6 in Chapter 4, and patients with other nonspecific types of arthritis have reported impressive improvement in arthritic symptoms when this treatment was administered for associated problems.

As an endocrinologist I do not encounter many patients with rheumatoid arthritis, but three additional patients with this diagnosis have been seen in recent years, and their responses to physiologic dosages of cortisone acetate or hydrocortisone have also been encouraging.

Case 1

The patient was a female, referred at age forty-six because of hypothyroidism associated with a goiter. Thyroid antibodies were present at a titer of 1:250 serum dilution, consistent with chronic thyroiditis, and she responded nicely to Euthroid, gr. 1½ daily, plus hydrocortisone, 5 mg four times daily. She also had a history of rheumatoid arthritis of twenty-five years duration, and when she was given the hydrocortisone for her thyroiditis, she reported significant improvement in symptoms of the rheumatoid arthritis. This improvement continued for over five years, during which time hydrocortisone was maintained at the same dosage except during respiratory infections, when it was temporarily doubled.

The coincidence of two autoimmune disorders, chronic thyroiditis and rheumatoid arthritis, in this patient was interesting and suggests some possible relationship. That low dosage glucocorticoid therapy administered for the thyroiditis also helped the arthritis strengthens this suspicion.

Case 2

The second patient (case number 2) was a female referred at the age of thirty-eight years because of irregular menses and occasional episodes of prolonged bleeding after her third and last pregnancy eight years previously. Four years prior to her referral, after a severe emotional upset, she developed pain and swelling in her fingers, ankles, and hips that was diagnosed as rheumatoid arthritis. Arthritic symptoms persisted until she was given hydrocortisone, 5 mg four times daily, for the menstrual disorder. They then improved impressively, with disappearance of joint swelling and only occasional mild pain. Her ovarian dysfunction required a combination of hydrocortisone, 5 mg four times daily, Euthroid, gr. 1 daily, and Premarin, 0.3 mg daily except during menses, for optimum benefit and resumption of ovulatory cycles, and on this therapy her arthritis has remained in remission for three years.

Case 3

The patient was a man with rheumatoid arthritis referred because of difficulty controlling his arthritic symptoms with glucocorticoid therapy. He was fifty-three years old and had had moderately severe rheumatoid arthritis for approximately twenty years, with a history of onset at the time of considerable stress at work. He had received gold injections but developed a reaction to these, so three years prior to his referral he had been started on "cortisone" injections at intervals of three to four weeks. In addition to the injections, he had been given prednisolone, 5 mg three times daily. Six months before his referral, injections had been discontinued and prednisolone dosage had been decreased to 5 mg twice daily. Motrin®, 400 mg four times daily, and Plaquenil®, 200 mg daily, had been added to his therapeutic program. His energy had been poor, and he had been sensitive to cold.

Physical examination revealed a thin male, with a height of 72 inches, weight of 149¾ pounds, and swollen, painful knees and ankles, who walked with difficulty using a cane. T_3 sponge uptake and T_4 were normal. After no prednisolone for over twenty-four hours, plasma cortisol at 8:45 AM was 11.2 μg%; after ACTH, this rose to 21.2 μg%.

It was therefore evident that he had maintained some adrenal responsiveness in spite of his glucocorticoid therapy, but the baseline plasma cortisol was low for the time of day at which it was drawn, and the response to ACTH was borderline. He had also been taking high potency vitamin and mineral supplements as well as "soya lecithin capsules," kelp, and large doses of Vitamin E. They were all tapered and discontinued except for a single supplementary multivitamin capsule daily. Prednisolone was discontinued, and hydrocortisone, 7.5 mg four times daily, was given in its place. Motrin was continued.

During the subsequent two and one-half years he has slowly improved, his arthritis becoming much better with only mild persistent discomfort and slight swelling of his ankles. He gained 25 pounds and is able to walk more comfortably. At times of respiratory infections and also at times of urinary tract infections, the dosage of hydrocortisone has been temporarily increased, but after recovery it was returned to 7.5 mg four times daily. Urinary infections were related to urologic problems, and these have been treated by a urologist.

These three cases are not dramatic, but they suggest a potential for physiologic dosages of glucocorticoids in rheumatoid arthritis, and the known safety of this type of therapy warrants its trial more extensively.

Another patient who demonstrated impressive benefit in symptoms of arthritis with a decrease in an elevated sedimentation rate to normal is Case 4.

Case 4

This female patient was referred to me at the age of thirty-two years because of repeated miscarriages. The menarche had occurred at age twelve, with regular menses every twenty-eight days, lasting four to five days. She had some acne, worse premenstrually, but no excessive hair growth. She was married at age twenty-two and had a full-term normal delivery two years later. Subsequently she had five successive miscarriages in a period of four years, all occurring at about the third month of gestation. She had been given estrogen and injections, probably progesterone, but no thyroid medication.

For the previous three or four years she had experienced intermittent discomfort in her legs and knees, worse after exercise, with occasional swelling and tenderness of the joints. She had also tended to tire easily and had little energy. She had experienced frequent respiratory infections all of her life. Some increase in pigmentation at the sides of her forehead and in some small scars on her extremities had been noted during the previous few months. Eczema had been present in childhood, and "growing pains" had occurred at age six. Her health had otherwise been good. She had no brothers or sisters. Her father had mild diabetes mellitus.

Physical examination revealed a slender but normally developed thirty-two year old female with normal skin texture. There was slight brownish pigmentation at the sides of the forehead and in the antecubital fossae. She had mild acne but no excessive hair growth. The thyroid was slightly enlarged, approximately one-and-one-half times normal size, diffuse, nontender, but slightly irregular. Breast development was normal with no masses. Height was 62 inches, weight was 103½ pounds with shoes, pulse 72 and regular, blood pressure 115/70. A soft systolic murmur was present at the cardiac apex. Knee joints were not enlarged or tender. A TSH test was normal, with normal baseline PBI and I^{131} uptake and normal response to TSH stimulation. Urinary 17-ketosteroids were 6.5 mg/24 hours, and cortisol metabolites (similar to 17-OHST) were 6.9 mg/24 hours, both well within normal limits. After 80 units of Acthar® Gel I.M., the 17-KS increased to 13.1 and cortisol metabolites to 36.5 mg/24 hours, consistent with normal adrenal responsiveness. Erythrocyte sedimentation rate was 30 mm/hour. Fractionation of urinary 17-KS revealed a low dehydroepiandosterone, a finding that had been observed in several patients with rheumatoid arthritis, so she was given prescriptions for Synthroid, 0.1 mg daily, and cortisone acetate, 2.5 mg four times daily. On this therapy she reported marked symptomatic improvement with rare joint discomfort. Her thyroid was still slightly enlarged, so the Synthroid dosage was increased to 0.15 mg daily. Her sedimentation rate decreased to 10 mm/hour. On several occasions when she discontinued the cortisone, joint pains and swelling returned, then subsided when medication was resumed.

After having been on this program for two years, she decided to try another pregnancy. After conception, the dosage of Synthroid was increased to 0.3 mg daily, the dosage of cortisone being continued at 2.5 mg four times daily throughout her pregnancy, which was uneventful and went to term with a normal delivery of a baby boy. She decided not to nurse her infant, and she felt so well that she took the cortisone quite irregularly for several months. Arthritic symptoms again returned, so she resumed the dosage of 2.5 mg four times daily with relief. After delivery the dosage of Synthroid was returned to 0.15 mg daily.

Six months later arthritic symptoms returned while she was taking 2.5 mg four times daily. Erythrocyte sedimentation rate was normal (5 mm/hour). The dosage of cortisone acetate was increased to 5 mg every eight hours with slight improvement, but joint pains and swelling persisted. The dosage was therefore increased to 5 mg four times daily. On this dosage arthritic symptoms subsided and she felt quite well.

After four months the dosage was decreased to 5 mg every eight hours because of a tendency to nocturia, and she continued to feel well.

Two years later she had another pregnancy, during which she took Synthroid, 0.2 mg daily, and cortisone acetate, 5 mg every eight hours, and she had a full-term, normal delivery. She did not nurse this baby either, and the dosage of Synthroid was decreased to 0.1 mg daily post partum.

It was therefore evident that treatment with small doses of cortisone acetate and thyroxin enabled her to carry two pregnancies to term after having had five successive miscarriages. Her arthritic symptoms also seemed to be quite sensitive to the dosage of cortisone, being affected by very slight changes in dosage. Although her arthritis was not as severe as that of the previous three patients, the elevated sedimentation rate, joint swelling, and tendency to relapse whenever the dosage of cortisone was decreased suggested that it could be classified as rheumatoid arthritis.

A similar type of arthritis occurring in women around the age of menopause or later has been termed "polymyalgia rheumatica,"[4] and it has been reported to respond nicely to relatively small doses of prednisone or triamcinolone,[5] but these dosages were still two to five times stronger than the subreplacement dosages used for our patients. Rothermich[6] and Healey[4] have called attention to the advantages and relative safety of low dosages of corticosteroids in the treatment of arthritis, but their reassurances have not been widely accepted.

Observations on one of the patients summarized in our report of 1967[2] are of special interest because they suggest a possibility for preventing progression of rheumatoid arthritis if physiologic dosages of cortisone or hydrocortisone are initiated early in the course of the disease. For that reason they will be briefly reviewed here.

Case 5

This patient developed migratory pains in the hips, elbows, metatarsal, and temporomandibular joints at age thirteen shortly after the menarche. After she had been unable to attend school for over a month because of these pains, intensive studies in the hospital resulted in a diagnosis of "probable rheumatoid arthritis," according to the criteria of the American Rheumatism Association.[7] The administration of cortisone acetate, 5 mg four times daily, resulted in complete relief of pain and swelling in approximately two weeks, and she was able to return to school.

A month later the dosage was reduced to 2.5 mg four times daily, and she remained asymptomatic for four months. A recurrence of pain and swelling in the joints then occurred, so the dosage was returned to 5 mg four times daily. Subsequently, the dosage was decreased to 2.5 mg four times daily twice, but on both occasions joint pain and swelling recurred, once after a three-month interval and the second time after only a two-week interval, so she returned to 5 mg four times daily, a dosage upon which she remained asymptomatic. The menses, which had occurred at intervals of three to five weeks since the menarche, became regular at four-week intervals after cortisone therapy was started. Steroid studies revealed no evidence of a summation effect of the exogenously administered cortisone, nor was there evidence that the plasma cortisol exceeded the normal range at any time with this therapy, even when it was checked one hour after a morning dose, the interval at which the maximum rise in plasma cortisol levels would be expected.

Six months after cortisone therapy had been started a small, nontoxic enlargement of the thyroid gland was noted. The administration of triiodothyronine, 25 mcg daily, resulted in return of the thyroid gland to normal size.

The patient was married at age nineteen and had normal pregnancies at age twenty and twenty-two, cortisone and triiodothyronine therapy being continued through both. Arthritis has remained in remission when cortisone acetate dosage has been maintained at 5 mg four times daily. Three years ago her steroid therapy was changed to hydrocortisone, 2.5 mg four times daily. She was asymptomatic on this for several months, but intermittent arthritis symptoms again returned, so the dosage was increased to 5 mg four times daily. At age twenty-two latex fixation was positive, but erythrocyte sedimentation rate was normal (8 mm/hour, corrected). At age twenty-seven sedimentation rate and SMAC were normal, and an ACTH test revealed a baseline plasma cortisol at 9 AM of 28 μg/dl, rising to 35 μg/dl, consistent with low adrenal reserve.

This raised a question whether low adrenal reserve had been present since the onset of symptoms at age thirteen, or whether it had developed later. Observations in other patients indicate that prolonged administration of subreplacement dosages of cortisone acetate or hydrocortisone does not impair adrenal response, so it is unlikely that her treatment would have caused this. The response of urinary cortisol metabolites to ACTH at age thirteen was apparently normal, but this is a less sensitive measure of cortisol production. Hence, we are unable to answer this question definitely, but it seems likely that low adrenal reserve had been present since the onset of her illness.

This patient has been followed for fourteen years, from age thirteen to twenty-seven, during which she has continued low dosage glucocorticoid therapy, married, and had two normal pregnancies. While she took cortisone acetate or hydrocortisone in a dosage of 5 mg four times daily, her arthritis remained in remission, but whenever the dosage was reduced to 2.5 mg four times daily, symptoms eventually returned. Although the course of rheumatoid arthritis in young persons varies greatly,[8] the evidence that her arthritis relapsed whenever the dosage of cortisone was reduced suggests that the dosage of 5 mg cortisone acetate four times daily was preventing progression of her disease.

Most physicians treating rheumatoid arthritis have encountered patients whose symptoms can be maintained in a satisfactory remission on 15 or 20 mg of cortisone acetate daily, whereas withdrawal of the steroid is followed by recurrence or exacerbation. In several reviews of steroid therapy in rheumatoid arthritis, maintenance doses in this range are recommended, especially in women with cases of only moderate severity.[9-11]

The possibility that these dosages might act in any way other than as a summation effect has received little attention, however, and it has usually been implied that larger doses were necessary, at least initially. Therapeutic effectiveness of comparable small doses of prednisone (5 mg or less daily)[12, 13] or dexamethasone

(0.75 mg or less daily)[14] have been reported, but unless the predni-steroids or other derivatives of cortisone or hydrocortisone prove to have an advantage of longer duration of therapeutic effect with a resulting ability to use a schedule of less frequent doses, there would appear to be no reason to use them in this small dosage range. It is also possible that the derivatives might have undesirable side effects that are not encountered with the natural glucocorticoids at low dosage levels.

It therefore appears that therapeutic trials in a larger series of cases with initial doses of cortisone acetate or hydrocortisone in this range for at least fourteen days before considering an increase are warranted, as are further studies to determine the nature of the antirheumatic effects. These recommendations were made in 1967,[2] but they still apply today.

The evidence that small, physiologic dosages of cortisone acetate or hydrocortisone can benefit arthritis raises questions regarding the mechanism of antirheumatic effects. For many years it has been assumed that such effects depend upon production of an excess of steroid in the body, yet several observations suggest that this assumption may be incorrect.

For example, if the antirheumatic effect were primarily due to a summation effect, the greatest improvement should occur during the first two weeks of treatment, with a subsequent tendency to relapse. Instead, clinical experience indicates that maximum beneficial effects do not occur until approximately two weeks after treatment is started, and they persist while the steroid is continued and for variable lengths of time after its withdrawal. The delay in attainment of maximum antirheumatic effect coincides to some extent with the time required for the body to adjust to exogenous steroid and raises the question whether some aspect of the adjustment might be responsible for this effect. Boland and Headley,[15] early in their experience with cortisone therapy of rheumatoid arthritis, noted that maximum overall improvement usually occurred two or three weeks after treatment was started and was "more frequently noted at or near the end of the gradual dose reduction." The similarity of time interval with that observed with low dosage therapy is interesting and suggests that, even with larger doses, antirheumatic effect probably depends upon some factor other than hypercortisonism.

Although the beneficial effect of low dosage glucocorticoid therapy in arthritis may be due to its beneficial effect on autoimmune disorders, the mechanism of such beneficial effect remains to be explained. The possibility that an obscure abnormality of steroid metabolism contributes in some manner must be considered. Although relative deficiencies of excretion of DHA are not pathognomonic of rheumatoid arthritis, nevertheless our finding that all five cases of this disease studied had similar abnormalities and that their abnormalities were similar to those observed in patients with rheumatoid arthritis by Hill and Dempsey[3] is impressive. Of further interest in this regard is a report[16] that women destined to develop rheumatoid arthritis have subnormal fertility and a reduced menstrual span. It is tempting to speculate that the lowered fertility and the arthritis, both of which may improve with low dosage glucocorticoid therapy, may be related to some underlying and as yet unidentified abnormality of steroid metabolism, possibly related to autoimmune factors.

Further evidence pointing to this possibility is the remission in rheumatoid arthritis that characteristically occurs during pregnancy. Although it has been generally assumed that this results from the increased plasma hydrocortisone levels that are characteristic of pregnancy, that pregnant women do not develop signs or symptoms of hypercortisonism suggests that it is not an excessive level of hydrocortisone but some as yet unrecognized change in steroid metabolism that is responsible for the improvement in arthritic symptoms.

In view of these observations it seems more logical in the treatment of arthritics to continue safe, subreplacement dosages of cortisone acetate or hydrocortisone with temporary increases in times of stress than to withdraw steroid therapy completely. This would apply to patients who apparently achieve a complete remission as well as to those who experience only partial improvement. The practice of continuing some arthritic patients on prolonged therapy with relatively low doses of glucocorticoid is well established in most clinics, but this is done, for the most part, with apprehension and with the intention of ultimately withdrawing the steroid. Because of this philosophy, when a patient achieves a complete symptomatic remission, therapy is usually terminated to determine whether the remission will be maintained. Unfortunately, relapses often occur.

In addition to rheumatoid arthritis, other autoimmune collagen disorders such as disseminated lupus erythematosus, scleroderma, and polyarteritis nodosa might show favorable responses to persistent administration of small, physiologic dosages of cortisone acetate or hydrocortisone, but I have not had an opportunity to try this type of treatment in patients with these disorders.

If patients are experiencing a relatively severe exacerbation of any of these collagen disorders, the initial dosage of cortisone acetate or hydrocortisone probably should be greater to achieve a clinical remission more rapidly, but once the remission is achieved, the continuation of a physiologic dosage indefinitely might prove to have therapeutic advantages without harmful side effects. In other words, treatment of these disorders might be best if it were similar to treatment of adrenal insufficiency: in acute stages, large dosages may be necessary; later, small maintenance dosages may be preferable to discontinuing therapy altogether.

REFERENCES

1. Homburger F, Bonner CD: The treatment of Rauol Dufy's arthritis. *N Engl J Med 301*:669-673, 1979.
2. Jefferies WMcK: Low-dosage glucocorticoid therapy; An appraisal of its safety and mode of action in clinical disorders including rheumatoid arthritis. *Arch Intern Med 119*:265-278, 1967.
3. Hill SR, Dempsey H: Steroid excretion patterns in rheumatoid arthritis. In Mills LC, Moyer JH (Eds.): *Inflammation and Diseases of Connective Tissues.* Philadelphia, Saunders, 1961, p. 529.
4. Healey LA: Polymyalgia rheumatica. In Hollander JL, McCarty DJ (Eds.): *Arthritis and Allied Conditions,* 8th ed. Philadelphia, Lea and Febiger, 1972, pp 885-889.
5. Dailey MP, McCarty DJ: Polymyalgia rheumatic begins at 40. *Arch Int Med 139*:743-744, 1979.
6. Rothermich NO: Corticosteroid therapy in rheumatoid arthritis; criteria and results. *Postgrad Med 36*:117-128, 1964.

7. A committee of the American Rheumatism Association: 1958 Revision of Diagnostic Criteria for Rheumatoid Arthritis, *Arthritis Rheum 2:*16, 1959.

8. Borkin RE: The clinical course of rheumatoid arthritis. In Bunim JJ (Eds.): *Bulletin on Rheumatic Diseases III:* 19, 20, 1952.

9. Boland EW: Adrenal cortical steroids and some of their synthetic analogues in the treatment of rheumatoid arthritis. In Talbot JH, Lockie LM (Eds.): *Progress in Arthritis.* New York, Grune, 1958, p. 130.

10. Ensign DC, Sigler JW, Wilson GM, Jr: Steroids in rheumatoid arthritis. *Arch Intern Med 104:*949-958, 1959.

11. Slocumb CH: Cortisone and related steroids in the treatment of rheumatoid arthritis. *Med Clin North Am 45:*1209-1218, 1961.

12. Shuster S, Williams IA: Pituitary and adrenal function during administration of small doses of glucocorticoids. *Lancet 1:*674-678, 1961.

13. DeAndrade JR: Pituitary-adrenocortical reserve during corticosteroid therapy: A report on the methopyrapone test in ten patients taking long-continued small doses. *J Clin Endocrinol Metab 24:*261-262, 1964.

14. Cohen A, Goldman J, Kanenson WL, Turner R, Rose I: Treatment of rheumatoid arthritis with dexamethasone. *JAMA 174:*831-834, 1960.

15. Boland EW, Headley NE: Management of rheumatoid arthritis with smaller (maintenance) doses of cortisone acetate. *JAMA 144:*365-372, 1950.

16. Kay A, Bach F: Subfertility before and after the development of rheumatoid arthritis in women. *Ann Rheum Dis 24:*169-173, 1965.

Chapter 7

ALLERGIC DISORDERS

THE EFFECTIVENESS of large doses of glucocorticoids in the treatment of bronchial asthma and other acute allergic phenomena is well known, but the dosages employed are sufficient to cause hypercortisonism with its undesirable and hazardous side effects if they are continued as maintenance therapy. The use of prolonged glucocorticoid therapy in chronic allergies has, therefore, been discouraged.

With the knowledge that physiologic dosages of cortisone acetate or hydrocortisone may be continued indefinitely without harmful side effects, plus that a number of patients who were given physiologic dosages for other reasons have reported impressive symptomatic improvement in their allergic conditions, it would be advisable to determine whether administration of physiologic dosages for prolonged periods might be helpful in any chronic allergic disorder.

The rationale for this type of therapy is supported by the observation, mentioned in Chapter 4 in the discussion of low adrenal reserve, that many patients with allergies have abnormal ACTH tests, with evidence either of low adrenal reserve or of a low baseline plasma cortisol level. This suggests that allergies may be associated with an abnormality of adrenocortical function in the cases with low adrenal reserve, or of hypothalamic or pituitary function or of glucocorticoid transport in those with low baseline plasma cortisol levels.

A number of animal studies also support the rationale for this type of therapy in allergic rhinitis, allergic asthma, anaphylaxis, and some urticarias, the so-called "immediate-type" hypersensitivity disorders or Type I reactions of Coombs and Gell.[1] This type of allergy is characterized by increased levels of histamine in affected tissues, and administration of histamine can produce Type I allergic reactions. It has been demonstrated that adrenalectomy results in accumulation of histamine in tissues,[2] associated with a reduction of histaminase, the enzyme that

104

destroys histamine,[3] whereas administration of hydrocortisone restores histaminase activity and causes depletion of tissue histamine stores. Also, hydrocortisone has been reported to inhibit histidine decarboxylase, the enzyme responsible for conversion of histidine to histamine.[4] Hence, hydrocortisone inhibits the production and accumulation of an excess of histamine in tissues.

Recent studies[5] have shown that patients with extrinsic asthma have positive correlation between changes in peak expiratory flow, circulating epinephrine, and cyclic AMP and inverse correlation between expiratory flow and plasma histamine. Plasma cortisol reaches its lowest diurnal level four hours before the maximum level of plasma histamine and the minimum levels of the other measurements. Normal subjects showed circadian changes in epinephrine levels similar to those of asthmatics, but the nocturnal rise in plasma histamine in normals was only 1.5 MMOL/L compared with 14 MMOL/L in asthmatics. The reason for this difference was not clear.

Why persons with Type I allergic disorders should have an excess of histamine therefore is not known, but the observation that physiologic dosages of cortisone or hydrocortisone can produce symptomatic improvement suggests some fundamental disorder in this aspect of their immune response, and the evidence that many patients with allergic disorders have either low baseline plasma cortisol levels or low adrenal reserve suggests that a relative deficiency of hydrocortisone may be a contributing factor to the excess of histamine.

A recent report suggests another factor that may contribute to the development of allergic rhinitis and asthma. Venter and associates[6] identified autoantibodies to β_2-adrenergic receptors in the serum of one patient with allergic rhinitis and two patients with asthma. Such antibodies may provide a mechanism for β-adrenergic resistance at the receptor level.

Almost every patient who had allergies associated with disorders for which small dosages of cortisone acetate or of hydrocortisone were given reported improvement in the allergies during this therapy. The beneficial effect of a small dosage of hydrocortisone in a patient with chronic allergic rhinitis and sinusitis was mentioned in case 2 in Chapter 5. Another impressive example is a girl who experienced decrease in bronchial asthma while being treated with low dosage glucocorticoid therapy for other problems.

Case 1

This patient was referred by her pediatrician at the age of fourteen years because of symptoms of hypothyroidism. During the previous year she had become chronically fatigued, sensitive to cold, her skin had become dry, and she had developed constipation. The menarche had occurred eighteen months previously, and her cycles had been quite irregular with intervals up to six months, menses lasting ten to fourteen days. Her growth had slowed, and she had gained over ten pounds. Her schoolwork had continued to be excellent, however, with straight As on her report card. She also had a history of intermittent bronchial asthma since age five, with increased symptoms in the previous two years.

Examination revealed a height of 58 inches, weight 102¼ pounds, blood pressure 90/60, pulse 68 and regular. Her skin was cool. The thyroid gland was diffusely enlarged, approximately twice normal size, with normal texture. There was no lymphadenopathy. Breast development was normal. Reflexes were equal and hypoactive with slow relaxation of ankle jerk. T_3 sponge uptake and T_4 were both low; a thyroid antibody test was negative.

She was given Synthroid, 0.1 mg daily, with improvement in fatigue, sensitivity to cold, dry skin, and constipation over the next month, but her asthma became worse. An ACTH test revealed a baseline plasma cortisol of 15 mcg% at 10:15 AM; thirty minutes after an I.M. injection of 25 units of Cortrosyn, this rose to 29 mcg%.

Because of the presence of irregular menses and of a thyroid condition suggesting chronic lymphocytic thyroiditis, although her thyroid antibody test was negative, cortisone acetate, 5 mg four times daily, was added to her therapeutic program. She returned a month later reporting impressive improvement in all symptoms including the asthma. She had grown almost an inch, weight was 92 pounds, blood pressure 100/70, pulse 76 and regular. Basal temperature chart showed a normal 32 day ovulatory cycle.

Subsequently she has maintained an optimum thyroid state with Euthroid, gr. 1 twice daily, plus cortisone acetate, 5 mg four times daily. The thyroid has decreased almost to normal size, and her asthma has remained in remission except during several respiratory infections, which have responded to treatment more quickly than prior to cortisone therapy. During respiratory infections, cortisone acetate has been increased to as much as 20 mg four times daily, depending upon severity of the illness, and symptoms have cleared in less than a week with no recurrences, in contrast to previous respiratory infections that had been much more severe and lasted for several weeks. Whenever evidence of bacterial infection has been present, she has been given either penicillin or erythromycin in therapeutic dosages in addition to increasing the dosage of cortisone acetate and has experienced rapid improvement. The patient, her mother, and her pediatrician have all been impressed by her improvement since receiving the small dosage of cortisone acetate, which she has been taking for over a year.

In addition to numerous typical symptoms of hypothyroidism, this fourteen year old girl had irregular, prolonged menses and bronchial asthma. The presence of a goiter suggested a chronic thyroiditis even though thyroid antibodies were not detected. An ACTH test was borderline low, so there was no clear indication for cortisone therapy, yet it produced dramatic improvement in her asthma and her ability to recover from respiratory infections, as well as in her menstrual cycles.

Case 2 is that of another asthmatic who experienced impressive improvement on small doses of hydrocortisone.

Case 2

This woman was first seen at the age of sixty-three with asthma of ten years duration and chronic respiratory infections with sinusitis and fatigue for the previous two months. She had had a hysterectomy for fibroids at age thirty-five, having bled intermittently for two years. Her cycles had previously been normal and she had had three full-term pregnancies.

Temperature tolerance had been normal, bowels had been regular, and she never had any hot flashes. She had been given injections for her asthma, but she had received no estrogen therapy. Increased hair growth on her chin had been noted for the previous five years. Six years previously a nodule in the thyroid had been removed, but no thyroid medication had been given. Her mother and sister had had goiters removed.

Physical examination revealed moderate hirsutism of the face, periareolar and subumbilical areas, and extremities. She had a residual suntan in February from the previous summer. Weight was 138¼ pounds, blood pressure 138/74, pulse 84 and regular. The thyroid scar was well healed, and there was no thyroid tissue palpable in the neck. Bilateral wheezes but no rales were present over both lungs. The liver edge was palpable, one finger-breadth below the right costal margin, not tender. T_3 sponge uptake was 41 percent, and T_4 was 10.2 mcg%. Urinary 17-KS were 7.0 mg/24 hours, and 17-OHST 8.2 mg/24 hours. Plasma cortisol at 8 AM was 10.0 mcg%; and an hour after an I.M. injection of 25 units of ACTH this rose to 45.0 mcg%. She volunteered that her asthma improved for four days after the ACTH test. She was therefore given a trial of Cortef, 5 mg four times daily.

She returned a month later reporting impressive improvement in her asthmatic symptoms, with less wheezing, better energy, and better appetite. After this improvement had been maintained for six months, the dosage was decreased to 2.5 mg four times daily. Shortly after the decrease she developed a mild respiratory infection, and her symptoms of asthma became worse, so a dosage of 5 mg four times daily was resumed, and she continued to take this dosage. Meanwhile, her liver edge became no longer palpable. In the spring of 1976 she had no respiratory infections or influenza, although most of the other workers at her place of employment were sick in an influenza epidemic.

Three months later the Cortef dosage was decreased to 5 mg before each meal and 2.5 mg at bedtime, and a week later she developed symptoms of pneumonia with a recurrence of bronchitis. This responded to antibiotics plus Marax®. Six months later she had a recurrence of asthmatic bronchitis that responded to predisone, 5 mg four times daily, and aminophyllin.

Cortef was resumed at 5 mg four times daily. Prednisone dosage was tapered and discontinued, and she has felt quite well for the subsequent two years. It was apparent that this patient was healthier on 5 mg Cortef four times daily than on any smaller dosage.

Observations such as these suggest that patients with chronic severe allergies should have therapeutic trials with prolonged courses of physiologic dosages of cortisone acetate or hydrocortisone, and shorter courses may be helpful in treating seasonal allergies. As with patients receiving subreplacement dosages for other conditions, at times of increased stress such as infections the dosage of cortisone acetate or hydrocortisone should be increased for the duration of the stress, then returned to the maintenance level. Such a therapeutic program may provide better control of the allergic condition and less need for other medications without causing a risk of hazardous side effects.

REFERENCES

1. Coombs RRA, Gell PGH: Classification of allergic reactions responsible for clinical hypersensitivity and disease. In Gell PGH, Coombs RRA (Eds.): *Clinical Aspects of Immunology.* Philadelphia. Davis Co, 1968, pp 575-596.
2. Halpern BN, Benacerraf B, Briot M: Roles of cortisone, desoxycorticosterone, and adrenaline in protecting adrenalectomized animals against hemorrhagic, traumatic, and histaminic shock. *Br J Pharmacol* 7:287-297, 1952.

3. Haeger K, Kahlson G, Westling H: Evidence of a regulatory mechanism controlling the levels of histamine and histaminase in the gastrointestinal tract. *Acta Physiol Scand (Suppl 111) 30:*177-191, 1953.

4. Slonecker CE, Lim WC: Effects of hydrocortisone on the cells in an acute inflammatory exudate. *Lab Invest 27:*123-128, 1972.

5. Barnes P, Fitzgerald G, Brown M, Dollery C: Nocturnal asthma and changes in circulating epinephrine, histamine, and cortisol. *N Engl J Med 303:*263-267, 1980.

6. Venter JC, Fraser CM, Harrison LC: Autoantibodies to B_2-adrenergic receptors: A possible cause of adrenergic hyporesponsiveness in allergic rhinitis and asthma. *Science 207:*1361-1363, 1980.

Chapter 8

OTHER AUTOIMMUNE DISORDERS

For many years it has been known that allergies are disorders of the immune response, but only recently has it been recognized that rheumatoid arthritis and other collagen diseases are associated with a disturbance of the immune system, wherein the body develops antibodies or immune complexes that damage some of its own tissues. With recent advances in the techniques for recognizing disorders of the immune mechanism, a number of other clinical conditions have been found to be associated with autoimmune phenomena. These include hyperthyroidism with diffuse goiter (Graves' disease), chronic lymphocytic thyroiditis (struma lymphomatosa), diabetes mellitus, regional enteritis, and ulcerative colitis. The possibility of beneficial effects of physiologic dosages of glucocorticoids has been suggested in each of these prior to the demonstration of their autoimmune basis, so now it is even more desirable to determine the potential contribution of this therapy in their management.

HYPERTHYROIDISM WITH DIFFUSE GOITER

In 1930 Marine[1] postulated that Graves' disease was associated with adrenocortical insufficiency. Both conditions are characterized by enlargement of the lymph nodes associated with a relative lymphocytosis. When cortisone first became available, it is not surprising that therapeutic trials of its administration to patients with this disorder were made. Hill, Reiss, Forsham, and Thorn in 1950[2] reported that cortisone acetate, in doses of 100 to 200 mg per day for sixteen days, produced a decrease in serum protein-bound iodine and basal metabolic rate in a patient with Graves' disease. This group also reported that "following an initial exacerbation of clinical hyperthyroidism (manifested chiefly by an increase in basal metabolic rate) both ACTH and cortisone appear to suppress thyroid function in about one half of the patients with Graves' disease in this limited series."

110

The clinical improvement in one patient given ACTH was so impressive that a subtotal thyroidectomy was performed with no other antithyroid medication!

In 1951 Rawson[3] stated that the adrenals of some hyperthyroid patients were not normally responsive to ACTH, and Lerman[4] stated that with tests of adrenal function available at that time, patients with Graves' disease appeared to have lowered adrenocortical function with inadequate response to stress.

Wikholm and Einhorn[5] in 1963 reported that 60 mg prednisolone daily for seven days to patients with hyperthyroidism produced a significant decrease in I^{131} uptake and an impressive decrease in serum protein-bound iodine. In 1964 Snyder, Green, and Solomon[6] reported that prednisone in doses of 40 to 60 mg daily resulted in disappearance of long-acting thyroid stimulator (LATS) from the serum of two patients with ophthalmopathic Graves' disease.

Such dosages are too large to be tolerated for extended periods, but the observations suggested that glucocorticoids may have a beneficial effect upon Graves' disease. With more recent evidence that LATS is an abnormal immune globulin, Graves' disease has become classified as an autoimmune disorder. Although it is not known why glucocorticoids are beneficial in autoimmune disorders or why larger dosages are required to produce beneficial effects in some cases than in others, the supplementation of antithyroid therapy with safe, physiologic dosages of cortisone acetate or hydrocortisone warrants study.

Favorable effects of pharmacologic dosages of cortisone in patients with thyroid storm[7] or with severe ophthalmopathy associated with Graves' disease[8] were also reported. These disorders are rare complications of Graves' disease, but glucocorticoid therapy has remained a valuable adjunct in their therapy. As with other severe disorders, initial dosages have been relatively high. The observations of Brown and his associates[8] indicate that large dosages are necessary to produce a remission in severe ophthalmopathy. Continuation of such dosages may produce serious side effects, however, yet when they are tapered and withdrawn altogether, relapses often occur. As soon as the ophthalmopathy has been brought under control, therefore, dosages for our patients have been reduced to physiologic levels and have been continued for months or even years. Such patients seemed to maintain remissions better and have fewer relapses than those who discontinued the steroid altogether. The advisability of administering small dosages of cortisone acetate or hydrocortisone to patients with Graves' disease without severe ophthalmopathy was therefore considered, and routine ambulatory ACTH tests on patients with this disorder were initiated.

As a consulting endocrinologist I do not see many cases of uncomplicated Graves' disease, since most of these are treated satisfactorily by primary care physicians. Hence, the cases referred to me have tended to be more complicated therapeutic problems. Although I have not had sufficient clinical experience to draw firm conclusions regarding this modification of therapy, patients who have received it have reported improvement in energy and a decrease in nervousness to a degree that warrants further investigation. An important question regarding its possible advantage is whether it improves the percentage of patients receiving permanent remissions from customary medical therapy.

A patient who exemplifies the value and safety of this type of therapy in moderately severe ophthalmopathy and pretibial myxedema was referred to me at the age of thirty-nine years because of exophthalmos.

Case 1

The patient had been married at age twenty-eight and had a full-term, normal delivery ten months later. Subsequently she had seven successive miscarriages, three in the first trimester and four at approximately six months gestation. During her fourth pregnancy, at age thirty-five, she developed hyperthyroidism and was treated with propylthiouracil and a subtotal thyroidectomy. Subsequently she developed hypothyroidism, and thyroid medication in doses up to gr. 6 daily had been given with some improvement. During this time she developed exophthalmos and marked swelling and thickening of the skin of the left leg and slight swelling and thickening of the skin of the right leg. At age thirty-seven her thyroid medication had been changed to Cytomel®, 100 mcg daily. She continued to be sensitive to both heat and cold; her hands and feet would get cold easily, but she perspired rather heavily.

Physical examination revealed no tremor; blood pressure was 112/85, pulse 92 and regular, weight 134 pounds, height 66½ inches without shoes. There was bilateral puffiness of the periorbital tissues, with marked lid retraction and slight chemosis of the bulbar conjunctivae. Extraocular movements were within normal limits except for slight diplopia on looking far to the right. Exophthalmometer readings were 26 mm on the right and 25 mm on the left. The thyroid was not palpable. Severe pretibial myxedema was present on the left leg with much brownish discoloration and induration, and mild pretibial myxedema on the right leg. A thyroidectomy scar was present but not pigmented. Serum PBI was 1.6 mcg/100 ml, and cholesterol was 127 mg per 100 cc. Urinary 17-KS were 10.0 mg and cortisol metabolites 9.9 mg/24 hours.

The PBI and cholesterol were consistent with an excessive dosage of triiodothyronine, since this medication does not contribute to serum PBI, and her exophthalmos and thyroid status improved after a decrease to 12.5 mcg of Cytomel twice daily plus 0.15 mg daily of Synthroid. Exophthalmometer measurements decreased to 24 mm bilaterally, but pretibial myxedema did not improve until prednisolone, 2.5 mg four times daily was added. On this regimen the pretibial myxedema improved progressively. A year later she conceived again. PBI was only 3.6 mcg%, so the dosage of thyroxine was increased to 0.3 mg per day. PBI then increased to 10.5 mcg%. At six months gestation the dosage of prednisolone was decreased to 1 mg four times daily. On this program she had a full-term delivery of a normal infant by Caesarean section. After delivery thyroxine dosage returned to 0.15 mg daily, and nine months later the steroid was changed to cortisone acetate, 5 mg four times daily.

The patient has subsequently been followed at intervals up to the present, seventeen years since she was first seen. Her thyroid status has remained stable, her exophthalmos has improved, with exophthalmometer readings remaining between 24 and 25 mm bilaterally, and her pretibial myxedema has cleared completely. Her present medications consist of Euthroid, gr. ½ twice daily, and Cortef, 5 mg four times daily. An ACTH test six months ago revealed a baseline plasma cortisol at 10:30 AM of 19 μg/dl; thirty minutes after an I.M. injection of 25 units of Cortrosyn this rose to 30 μg/dl. Two years ago plasma cortisol at 2 PM was 6.6 μg%; thirty minutes after an I.M. injection of 25 units of Cortrosyn this rose to 19 μg%.

Although ophthalmopathy and pretibial myxedema apparently developed while the patient had postoperative hypothyroidism, it was evident that excessive replacement with triiodothyronine did not help and may have aggravated this complication. Subsequent improvement in ophthalmopathy and clearing of pretibial myxedema with smaller dosages of thyroid medications plus physiologic dosages of glucocorticoid was impressive, and her successful full-term, normal pregnancy after having had seven successive miscarriages indicated that her general hormonal status had improved.

Case 2 also demonstrates the beneficial long-term effects of low doses of hydrocortisone in ophthalmopathy associated with Graves' disease, but the patient is, in addition, an example of several other problems worthy of comment.

Case 2

This fifty-six year old female was referred because of an eye problem. Two years previously she had developed redness and irritation of both eyes. She had been taking Aldomet® for high blood pressure for four years, but her health had otherwise been good. A physician had told her the inflammation was probably due to an infection, and she was given drops which she used for two months without benefit. Four months later she was admitted to a hospital for studies, and tests suggested mild hyperthyroidism. She was given propylthiouracil, 200 mg four times daily, plus Diuril® and Valium®. Aldomet was continued.

After taking the propylthiouracil for six months, she was admitted to another hospital by a different physician, who had her stop all previous medications for three months. During this time her eyes became much worse, with more prominence and inflammation. She had then been given large doses of prednisone, which were subsequently tapered and discontinued three months later. A scan was performed, and she was told that her thyroid was normal. Three months later an ophthalmologist performed a decompression operation on both orbits, followed in four months by a muscle resection for diplopia. Prednisone, 25 mg every other day for a week, then nothing for a week, was administered for six weeks. She was then referred to me. At the time of referral she was taking only Aldomet, one tablet daily.

She had been sensitive to heat all her life. At age twelve she was told she had "a tendency to a goiter." She also noted occasional diarrhea. Eighteen months before referral she sometimes felt "trembly," and her appetite was "too good." She gained 30 pounds with prednisone treatment, her usual weight being 140 pounds. Arthritic pains in her hands and sacroiliac area were relieved with the prednisone, but this therapy caused extreme weakness.

Past history included severe pneumonia at nine months of age, many "bronchial troubles," and a tendency to catch colds that settled in her chest. A cholecystectomy for stones was performed at age forty-one. The menarche occurred at age twelve, cycles had been regular, but she had much dysmenorrhea. She had only one pregnancy with a normal, full-term delivery. No further pregnancies occurred in spite of a lack of precautions. The menopause occurred at age forty-seven, with hot flashes for which she had received "hormone shots" every six weeks for several months. Family history was negative for thyroid disorders, but both parents had high blood pressure.

Physical examination revealed a height of 63½ inches, weight 171 pounds, blood pressure 160/100, pulse 108 and regular. There was moderate periorbital puffiness and moderate injection of the sclera. Slight widening of the palpebral fissure was present on the left with diplopia in all directions except slightly below the horizontal. Extraocular movements of the right eye were within normal limits, but there was slight impairment of upward and lateral gaze with the left eye. Exophthalmometer readings were 30 mm on the right and 29 mm on the left eye. The thyroid was not definitely palpable. There was no tremor. T_3 sponge uptake was 59 percent. T_4 6.1 mcg%. Plasma cortisol at 8:45 AM was 33.0 μg/dl; thirty minutes after an I.M. injection of 25 units of Cortrosyn this rose to 45.5 μg/dl.

The patient was given saturated solution of potassium iodide, 5 drops daily, Cortef, 5 mg four times daily, Multicebrin®, 1 daily, and Euthroid, gr. ½ daily, and gradual improvement occurred. Blood pressures were in upper normal range, and Aldomet was discontinued without change. After two years of this therapy she continues to feel well, and she has had no further arthritic pains. Slight puffiness of the periorbital tissues persists with extraocular movements within normal limits. Diplopia is no longer present except on extreme upward gaze. Exophthalmometer readings are 24 mm bilaterally, blood pressure 160/90.

It is not unusual for the diagnosis of endocrine ophthalmopathy to be missed. Whenever a patient with a history of Graves' disease develops eye problems, it should be suspected, but when a patient with no history of thyroid disorder presents with inflammation of the eyes, it is certainly not the first diagnosis to be considered. Nevertheless, unless it is considered, much time may be lost. Even when it is suspected, other conditions such as conjunctivitis or tumor of the orbit should be ruled out. When the diagnosis is made, the use of propylthiouracil, especially in large dosages, may not be the best antithyroid therapy. Mild hyperthyroidism with ophthalmopathy seems to respond better to iodide, with the addition of thyroxine if the patient becomes hypothyroid.[7]

Propylthiouracil in the relatively large dosage of 200 mg four times daily should be reserved for patients with severe hyper-thyroidism, and I prefer to avoid the thiourea derivatives in patients with severe ophthalmopathy. Furthermore, although diuretics have been reported to be symptomatically helpful in severe exophthalmos, glucocorticoids are much more effective. The use of tranquilizers in hyperthyroidism also seems logical, but except for reserpine or propranolol in certain cases, other tranquilizers have not been very helpful.

The patient then sought advice from another physician, and he had her stop all previous medications for three months. This probably was unwise because not only is it more difficult to evaluate thyroid status after antithyroid drugs are withdrawn, but also relapses may occur more abruptly. It is better to study patients while they are on their previous therapeutic program, unless they are having a toxic reaction to a medication. Therapy can then be changed as indicated, but only relatively slowly. Rapid changes in endocrine therapy sometimes seem to cause additional problems, as occurred in this case.

The exacerbation of ophthalmopathy following withdrawal of medications was treated with large doses of prednisone with temporary improvement, but discontinuance of this therapy after three months was followed by another relapse that resulted in bilateral decompression operations. Such surgical procedures are advisable as last resort measures to prevent loss of sight, but if suitable medical therapy, including treatment with saturated solution of potassium iodide, glucocorticoids, and small doses of thyroxine or thyroxine plus triiodothyronine if hypothyroidism develops, is administered on a consistent, stable program, surgery rarely seems to be necessary.

The development of weakness on prednisone therapy suggests the development of hypokalemia, a relatively common complication of large dosages of glucocorticoids administered for prolonged periods. In my experience dosages of 20 mg prednisone daily may be needed in acute endocrine ophthal-mopathy, but they should be tapered as rapidly as possible as soon as the acute inflammatory state begins to subside.

Case 3
    A twenty-three year old female patient was referred by her ob-

stetrician in the third month of her first pregnancy because of hyper-thyroidism. For three months she had suffered increased nervousness, tremor, and a tendency to diarrhea. She had lost some weight, but this had been attributed to morning sickness. T_3 sponge uptake had been 39 percent, and T_4 had been greater than 13.0 mcg%. The menarche had occurred at age thirteen or fourteen; cycles had always been irregular with intervals of twenty-eight to sixty days, menses lasting seven days with a heavy flow and cramps. She had experienced severe headaches two days premenstrually.

Physical examination revealed slight widening of the palpebral fissures, moderate tremor, and a diffuse enlargement of the thyroid gland approximately one-and-one-half times normal size. Height was 60¾ inches, weight was 107¾ pounds, blood pressure 114/70, pulse 100 and regular. T_3 by RIA was 335 ng/ml (normal 90-200). A thyroid antibody test was negative.

A diagnosis of mild hyperthyroidism in the third month of pregnancy was made, and she was given a prescription for saturated solution of potassium iodide, 5 drops daily in milk. She returned a week later reporting some improvement in nervousness, but she was still chronically fatigued with much aching of her muscles, and she continued to have frequent nausea and vomiting. Weight was 109¼ with sandals, blood pressure 118/70, pulse 104 and regular. Moderate tremor, slight stare, and enlargement of the thyroid gland were unchanged. Plasma cortisol at 2 PM was 25 mcg%. Because of her history of irregular menses, cortisone acetate, 5 mg four times daily, was added to her therapeutic regimen. An antacid was administered with each dose of cortisone because of the nausea associated with pregnancy.

She returned two weeks later reporting some improvement, but she was still depressed and nervous, with much nausea and insomnia. Tremor was no longer present, weight was 114 pounds, blood pressure 110/60, pulse 80 and regular. T_4 was 8.3 mcg%.

A month later she returned feeling much better; nausea had subsided, nerves were calm, and she was sleeping well.

The remainder of her pregnancy was normal and uneventful. The potassium iodide was discontinued six weeks before delivery, but cortisone acetate was continued up to delivery, which was performed by Caesarean section because of a narrow pelvic outlet. No supplementary glucocorticoid was given at the time of her Caesarean section, which she tolerated well.

She chose not to nurse her baby. Cortisone acetate and potassium iodide were resumed when she was able to take oral medication post partum. Six weeks post partum her obstetrician had her start an oral contraceptive. She has no complaints six months later. Her thyroid has increased slightly to approximately two-and-one-half times normal size, but she has no other signs or symptoms of thyroid disorder, weight being 113½ pounds with shoes, blood pressure 110/70, pulse 76 and regular. Potassium iodide will be discontinued soon, and if her condition remains stable, cortisone acetate will also be discontinued.

Because of her history of menstrual irregularity, an ACTH test will be performed after cortisone acetate has been discontinued, and if her cycles become irregular again, this medication will be resumed.

Although this patient might have improved as well on potassium iodide therapy alone, her initial response to iodide treatment was poor, the administration of cortisone acetate was followed by progressive improvement with a full-term delivery of a normal baby, and her thyroid status has remained stable post partum.

Although antithyroid drugs such as propylthiouracil or methimazole (Tapazole®) may be used safely to treat hyperthyroidism during pregnancy, provided proper care is taken to avoid excessive suppression of the thyroid, saturated solution of potassium iodide is still a good therapy for this type of problem, and it avoids the danger of side effects of the thiourea drugs. Because patients with ovarian dysfunction often have their disorder become worse after oral contraceptives, I prefer to avoid their use in such cases, but occasionally the risk of another pregnancy may be sufficiently great and the likelihood of adequate protection by other contraceptive measures sufficiently uncertain so as to justify them as the lesser of two evils.

CHRONIC THYROIDITIS

A related disorder in which physiologic dosages of glucocorticoids have therapeutic promise is chronic thyroiditis. This not only applies to chronic lymphocytic thyroiditis, or struma lymphomatosa, which appears to be etiologically related to Graves' disease, but also to at least some other types of chronic thyroiditis. Yamada and his associates[9] have reported beneficial effects of 1 mg dexamethasone orally twice daily in patients with struma lymphomatosa.

An example of the beneficial effects of low dosage glucocorticoid therapy in nonspecific thyroiditis is case 4.

Case 4
This thirty-two year old female was referred because of a thyroid

problem. Nine months previously she had an attack of "flu" during which her thyroid became swollen and tender and her face became puffy. T_4 was 3.5 mcg% and I^{131} uptake 53 percent, with diffuse enlargement of her thyroid gland. She was given Synthroid, 0.025 mg daily for five months. On this treatment her T_4 was 2.0 mcg%. The Synthroid was then discontinued, and she developed progressive sluggishness and sensitivity to cold. She had suffered from bronchial asthma as long as she could remember, for which she had received Quadrinal® and injections of Aristocort® Forte. Her energy had also been poor as long as she could remember. The menarche had occurred at age twelve, with regular cycles, menses lasting from five to six days. She was married and had two children.

Physical examination revealed a height of 61¾ inches, weight 107 pounds, blood pressure 90/60, pulse 88 and regular. Her hands and feet were cold, and her voice was slightly hoarse. The thyroid was diffusely enlarged two-and-one-half times normal size, not tender. There was no lymphadenopathy. Moderate chronic cystic mastitis was present bilaterally. There was no acne or hirsutism. A thyroid antibody test was negative. T_3 sponge uptake was 40 percent; T_4 was less than 1.0 mcg%. Sedimentation rate was 8 mm/hour, hematocrit 39 percent. Plasma cortisol at 2 PM was 12.2 µg%; thirty minutes after an I.M. injection of 25 units of ACTH, this rose to 32.8 µg%.

A diagnosis of hypothyroidism with goiter, possibly due to a previous thyroiditis, was made. On Synthroid, 0.15 mg daily, and cortisone acetate, 5 mg four times daily, she had a gradual but dramatic improvement in all of her symptoms, including the bronchial asthma, and her thyroid returned to normal size. Thickening of glandular tissue in the breasts also cleared.

Case 1 in Chapter 6 is an example of the beneficial effect of a subreplacement dosage of hydrocortisone on chronic thyroiditis.

DIABETES MELLITUS

Another condition in which physiologic dosages of hydrocortisone appear to have therapeutic benefit is diabetes mellitus. This undoubtedly would come as a surprise to many, because a characteristic effect of excessive dosages of glucocorticoid in diabetics is an increase in blood sugar levels and an increased requirement for insulin. Yet, a number of patients with diabetes mellitus experience marked fluctuations in blood sugar levels with swings from hyperglycemia to hypoglycemia, resulting in difficulty of control and much clinical distress. The ultimate manifestation of this disorder of labile diabetes mellitus is seen in patients with both diabetes mellitus and adrenal insufficiency.[10] where the body's mechanisms for protection against both high and low levels of blood sugar are impaired. Although epinephrine, glucagon, and growth hormone also help to protect against hypoglycemia, the presence of adequate levels of glucocorticoid seems to be of primary importance, since in adrenal insufficiency the endogenous supply of the other hormones does not prevent insulin hypersensitivity and hypoglycemia. The presence of chronic, low-grade infections can also cause lability in diabetics, so these conditions should be carefully ruled out.

Patients with labile diabetes mellitus are often young, active persons. They can be benefited to some extent by adjusting their food intake to times of increased exercise or maximum insulin effect, by adjusting their insulin dosage and schedule and by decreasing intake of caffeine, which depletes liver-glycogen, but sometimes these measures will not produce adequate control. In such cases, the administration of hydrocortisone, 5 mg four times daily, has been found to stabilize their condition and help prevent hypoglycemia. Because this dosage does not result in hypercortisonism, it does not cause an increase in insulin requirement; on the contrary, it may result in a decrease in insulin dosage. These patients almost invariably have said that they feel better, with more energy and less fatigue, while taking the steroid.

Routine ACTH tests often show evidence of low adrenal reserve in such cases, but in others, ACTH tests may fall within normal limits. It is interesting to note that the incidence of diabetes mellitus in patients with Addison's disease is more than double that for the general clinic population, and recent evidence that both of these conditions may result from autoimmune phenomena probably explains this occurrence.

It has been our policy for a number of years to treat patients with labile diabetes with small doses of hydrocortisone, but the recent reports of evidence that diabetes mellitus may be a manifestation of an autoimmune process[11, 12] raises the question whether other patients with diabetes mellitus might benefit from such therapy. Although the mechanism of action of glucocorticoids in autoimmune processes is not understood, the beneficial therapeutic effect of glucocorticoids in patients with autoimmune disorders is well documented.

Another type of diabetic that has shown impressive improvement with physiologic dosages of cortisone acetate or hydrocortisone is the patient with insulin resistance. When such patients are given physiologic dosages of one of these steroids, insulin requirement frequently decreases impressively, and the patients experience striking improvement in energy and sense of wellbeing.

REGIONAL ENTERITIS, ULCERATIVE COLITIS, AND MUCOUS COLITIS

These are three other clinical conditions in which glucocorticoid therapy has been beneficial, and the demonstration that they may be related to autoimmune phenomena possibly explains this beneficial action. The apprehension associated with the employment of these agents, however, has discouraged their use in many clinics. Yet, numerous patients can be maintained in remission by taking small, physiologic dosages of cortisone acetate or hydrocortisone, whereas an exacerbation occurs if the steroid is discontinued. Dr. Crohn, who originally described regional ileitis and granulomatous colitis and who has seen more than 2,000 cases, states,[13] "My experience is that 90 percent of patients can be managed with medication, diet, and rest, and that only 10 percent require surgery. I give moderate doses of prednisone — usually starting with 15 mg a day and cutting down to 10 mg and then to 5 mg . . . I have had no problem with serious side effects even with long term therapy." The 5 mg prednisone he administers is equivalent to 20 mg hydrocortisone. Investigation of the use of prolonged maintenance therapy with subreplacement dosages in these disorders, therefore, certainly seems warranted.

It is interesting to note that Dr. Crohn further states, "The patients soon learn to adjust their own therapy in accordance with their needs. In the case of fever or acute exacerbation, I give an injection of hydrocortisone sodium succinate. . . . " This adjustment of dosage is consistent with the larger dosage necessary to maintain a patient with adrenal insufficiency in optimum health during periods of increased stress and is consistent with the principle that because hormone requirements may fluctuate, optimum hormone therapy may require variation in dosage under different circumstances.

Patients with mucous colitis or irritable bowel syndrome, conditions that may also have an allergic basis, have also reported impressive improvement during low dosage glucocorticoid therapy, so this type of treatment should be further investigated in these disorders.

REFERENCES

1. Marine D: Remarks on the pathogenesis of Graves' disease. *Am J Med Sci 180:*767-772, 1930.
2. Hill SR, Jr., Reiss RS, Forsham PH, Thorn GW: The effect of adrenocorticotropin and cortisone on thyroid function: Thyroid-adrenocortical interrelationships. *J Clin Endocrinol 10:*1375-1400, 1950.
3. Rawson RW in discussion of Wolfson WQ, Beierwaltes WH, Robinson WD, Duff IF, Jones JR, Knorpp CT, Siemienski JS, Eya M: Corticogenic hypothyroidism: Its coincidence, clinical significance and management during prolonged treatment with ACTH and cortisone. In Mote JR (Ed.): *Proceedings of Second Clinical ACTH Conference*, Vol. 2. Philadelphia, Blakiston, 1951, p. 95.
4. Lerman J; In Werner SC (Ed.): *The Thyroid*. New York, Hoeber, 1955, p. 598.
5. Wikholm G, Einhorn J: Effect of prednisolone and triiodothyronine on thyroid function in hyperthyroidism. *J Clin Endocrinol Metab 23:*76-80, 1963.
6. Snyder NJ, Green DE, Solomon DH: Glucocorticoid-induced disappearance of long-acting thyroid stimulator in the ophthalmopathy of Graves' disease. *J Clin Endocrinol Metab 24:*1129-1135, 1964.
7. Jefferies WMcK: Treatment of exophthalmos from the viewpoint of an internist. *AMA Arch Ophthalmol 56:*671-677, 1956.
8. Brown J, Coburn JW, Wigod RA, Hiss JM, Jr., Dowling JT: Adrenal steroid therapy of severe infiltrative ophthalmopathy of Graves' disease. *Am J Med 34:*786-95, 1963.
9. Yamada T, Ikejiri K, Kotani M, Kusakabe T: An increase of plasma triiodothyronine and thyroxine after administration of dexamethasone to hypothyroid patients with Hashimoto's thyroiditis. *J Clin Endocrinol Metab 46:*784-790, 1978.
10. Gowen WM: Addison's disease with diabetes mellitus. *N Engl J Med 61:*43-51, 1932.

11. Freitag G, Kloppel G: Insulinitis — a morphologic review. *Curr Top Pathol* *58:*49-90, 1973.
12. Craighead JE: Current views on the etiology of insulin-dependent diabetes mellitus. *N Engl J Med 299:*1439-1445, 1978.
13. Crohn B: (quoted in) *Medical World News,* August 2, 1974, p. 36.

Chapter 9

RESPIRATORY INFECTIONS

THE COMMON COLD

BEFORE CORTISONE became available, patients with chronic adrenal insufficiency were extremely vulnerable to stresses of any kind, and an ordinary respiratory infection often caused an acute collapse that was termed an "adrenal crisis." Patients had to be taken to a hospital and given intravenous saline and glucose as well as a parenteral adrenal cortical extract if that were available. After cortisone and hydrocortisone were introduced, patients with Addison's disease were still cautioned regarding respiratory illness, and they were instructed that upon developing the initial symptoms of a common cold they should increase the dosage of glucocorticoid and phone their physician immediately. Concern regarding the occurrence of respiratory illness in such patients was enhanced by the knowledge that large doses of glucocorticoids could impair resistance to infection while masking the symptoms.[1]

It was, therefore, a finding of some surprise and considerable relief that months and then years passed with patients consistently reporting that they had either no common colds or only very mild attacks. Most patients had no symptoms even suggestive of these disorders, but when symptoms did occur, a prompt increase in the dosage of glucocorticoid was often followed by a disappearance of symptoms without recurrence when the dosage was returned to maintenance levels. During this time, other members of the patients' families seemed to have their usual quota of respiratory illnesses, so the absence of such illness in the patients could not be attributed to lack of exposure to the viruses.

An additional reassuring observation was that when patients with adrenal insufficiency developed respiratory infections, the increase in dosage of replacement glucocorticoid did not cause an increase in complicating bacterial infections such as sinusitis

124

or bronchitis, and unless a bacterial complication developed, antibiotic therapy was not necessary.

The question naturally was raised whether the patients who apparently experienced shortened or aborted courses were really developing respiratory illness, but when a number of patients reported the same phenomenon at times when other members of their families were having acute respiratory illnesses, it appeared that the increase in dosage of glucocorticoid at the onset of the infection might be enabling the patient either to ward off or to recover from the infection more quickly. This possibility did not seem too unreasonable, since the development of common colds or other upper respiratory illnesses is often related to a "decrease in resistance" on the part of the host. The various conditions that seem to decrease resistance, such as excessive fatigue, lack of sleep, and emotional upsets, are those that would throw more strain on the hypothalamic-pituitary-adrenal system.

Meanwhile, patients who were receiving physiologic dosages of glucocorticoids for other conditions such as hirsutism or ovarian dysfunction began to report that they seemed to get fewer colds than other members of their families, often escaping completely when everyone else in the family had been ill. Every patient on low dosage glucocorticoid therapy did not report this apparent protective effect, but many did.

The possibility that glucocorticoids might enhance resistance to infection is so contrary to their well-known effect of impairing immunity that it was initially considered with skepticism. Yet, a review of the medical literature reveals an impressive amount of evidence that physiologic amounts of glucocorticoids can have a protective effect against infection. Perla and Marmorston summarized the evidence for this effect prior to 1941,[2] and Beisel and Rapoport summarized this evidence up to 1969.[3]

Both morphologic and physiologic studies point to a significant role of the adrenal glands in the defense mechanism of the body against intoxications and infectious diseases. In the 1920s Aschoff[4] and Goldzieher[5] described striking morphologic changes in the adrenals in infectious diseases. Infections such as diphtheria, scarlet fever, and every septic condition observed during World War I, including streptococcal infections and infections due to gas bacillus, were associated with marked edema of the adrenal cortex and diffuse regression of lipoid material. Fatal cases of malaria and peritonitis were also reported to have evidence of degeneration and necrosis in the adrenal cortex, with hemorrhage and arterial thromboses, without similar changes in other organs. Acute hemorrhagic necrosis of the adrenal cortices in some cases of meningitis, so-called Waterhouse-Friderichsen syndrome, is well known, and a less severe but life-threatening reversible adrenal insufficiency has been reported in fulminant meningococcemia.[6]

With evidence that the adrenals may be seriously damaged in the course of severe infections, the question arose whether the cortex or the medulla was primarily involved in resistance to infection. In 1926 Jaffe and Plavska,[7] in studies of susceptibility of adrenalectomized rats to typhoid vaccine, noted that evidence strongly suggested the greater significance of the cortex than of the medulla. Dr. David Marine, who performed classical research on the relationship of iodine deficiency to development of goiter, also studied the relationship of the adrenals to resistance.[8] Ingle[9] confirmed the observation that the cortex was more important in maintaining the resistance of the organism to histamine shock. Hartman and Scott[10] and Perla[11] determined that adrenocortical extract raised the resistance of adrenalectomized rats to typhoid vaccine almost to normal. Pottenger and Pottenger[12] reported that adrenocortical extract injections were beneficial in protecting guinea pigs against experimental tuberculosis infection. These investigators also reported that the administration of adrenocortical extract to tuberculous patients improved their energy and lessened fatigue. Whitehead and Smith[13] reported encouraging results of administration of injections of adrenal cortical extract to patients with severe infections such as typhoid fever, undulant fever, cellulitis, and sinusitis.

In 1941 Kendall reported that as little as 30 mcg of Compound E would protect an adrenalectomized rat against twenty-five minimum lethal doses of typhoid vaccine.[14] In 1954 Benedek and Montgomery[15] reported that patients with rheumatoid arthritis experienced fewer infections during 465 months of cortisone and/or ACTH therapy than during 411 months without such therapy. These were patients on various dosages of glucocorticoids! In 1958 Kass and Finland[16] reported that when adrenalectomized mice maintained with various replacement doses of cortisone were inoculated with pneumococci, survival was greatest in the groups whose maintenance dose most closely approximated normal adrenocortical status. By contrast, mortality increased progressively toward the extremes of either hypo- or hypercortisonism.

In 1960 Spink,[17] in a report of the use of adrenal steroids in patients with infectious diseases, stated, "Judicious use of corticotropin and other corticosteroids frequently contributed to immediate improvement in the condition of patients seriously ill with infections and their complications," and "An inventory of the (81) patients treated in this study has revealed no significant ill effects when the steroids were administered for only a few days, even when large doses were used."

In 1969 Beisel and Rapoport,[3] in a comprehensive review of interrelations between adrenocortical functions and infectious illness, stated "that the human host does fare best when his own pituitary-adrenal axis is normally responsive (or when exogenous hormone is given in optimal replacement dose after adrenalectomy) is a conclusion based upon extensive clinical data and well confirmed evidence in laboratory animals." They further stated that "present information suggests that the secretion of all major corticosteroid hormones is stimulated early in the course of acute infectious illness," and that "all available data support the concept that the glucocorticoid increase in the period of early symptoms varies in magnitude with the clinical severity of an infectious illness." It seems unlikely that nature would, at the onset of an infection, cause increased production of a hormone that would impair resistance to the infection. It is much more likely that the increased production of glucocorticoid serves to improve resistance in some fashion.

More recent reports provide more direct evidence that these steroids contribute in some fundamental fashion to normal immunity.

Ambrose[18] has presented evidence that a physiologic level of glucocorticoid is essential to the initiation of the immune process. Pierpaoli and Sorkin[19] state that the effect of the thymus upon the development of the immune mechanism appears to be mediated through the adrenals. Shakelford and Feigin,[20] in studies of the susceptibility of mice to pneumococcal infection, found that the longest survival was associated with maximal endogenous corticosterone response.

It is therefore evident that *physiologic* levels of glucocorticoids, in contrast to pharmacologic levels, have a fundamental *favorable* effect upon the body's resistance to infection.

Recent observations in our clinic seem to be pertinent to this point. Because so many patients reported apparent improvement in resistance to common respiratory infections while receiving physiologic subreplacement dosages of cortisone acetate or hydrocortisone, these dosages were given to patients who had histories of excessive susceptibility to respiratory infections. When they reported dramatic improvement in resistance to such infections, it was decided to study their circulating immune globulin levels, a method of measuring circulating antibodies that had just become available for clinical use. It was found that such patients frequently had relatively low circulating levels of IgM, the component that seems to be a primary factor in early response to viral and bacterial infections; the administration of 5 mg 4 times daily of cortisone acetate or hydrocortisone was accompanied by a rise not only in circulating levels of IgM but often also in levels of IgG and IgA (Fig. 6).[21] When the steroid was stopped, levels of immune globulins decreased, and susceptibility to respiratory infections returned. Hence, the improvement in resistance that occurs in such patients appears to be related to an increase in circulating immune globulins, especially IgM.

Several reports over the years have pertained to the effects of ACTH, adrenocortical hormone, and cortisone upon antibody production. Blanchard[22] in 1934 reported that administration of adrenocortical hormone to intact animals resulted after a period of ten days in a slight rise in opsonic power above the normal level. Fox and Whitehead[23] in 1935 reported that administration of cortical extract to adult normal rabbits and rats increased the production of hemolysins to sheep red blood cells from 40 percent to 70 percent higher than controls. White[24]

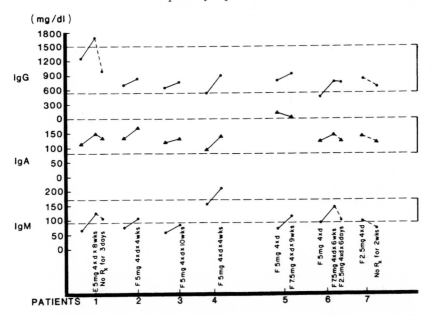

Figure 6. Effect of physiologic dosages of cortisone acetate (E) or cortisol (F) upon circulating levels of IgG, IgA, and IgM. Solid lines indicate effects of an increase in dosage, broken lines indicate effects of decrease in dosage. Horizontal interrupted lines indicate normal ranges for the technique employed.

in 1947 reported that cortisone and ACTH have a stimulating effect upon antibody production associated with an increase in the number and activity of phagocytic cells in lymphoid tissue and the dissolution of antibody-containing lymphocytes. Dougherty, Chase, and White[25] reported that administration of ACTH was followed by a rise in circulating antibody. These reports were soon forgotten, however, when numerous reports of the detrimental effect of cortisone and ACTH upon circulating antibody appeared. In retrospect, it seems likely that these discrepancies resulted from differences in dosages of ACTH and cortisone administered to experimental animals, those administered by White and his associates being physiologic, and those administered by others being pharmacologic. This certainly seems to be an explanation for the discrepancy between the report of Levy and Waldman[26] in 1974 that relatively large dosages of cortisol in mice decreased levels of IgG, IgA, and IgM and our findings that physiologic dosages increased levels of these immune globulins.

Identification of components of the immune response such as T-lymphocytes, B-lymphocytes, immunoglobulins, complement, and interferon has been advancing rapidly in recent years, but little is known about the factors that affect these components. Hence, further studies of the effects of physiologic versus pharmacologic dosages of glucocorticoids upon all of the components would be of interest. It appears that the increase in IgM with glucocorticoid therapy occurs chiefly in subjects with low circulating levels of this immune globulin, because subjects with normal levels may not show an increase, and subjects with high levels may even show a decrease during such treatment. Hence, this effect does not appear to be a general stimulatory one but rather to depend upon the initial state of the host.

It would also be of interest to determine the effects, if any, of other components of adrenocortical secretion, such as aldosterone, dehydroepiandrosterone, androstenedione and estrone, upon the immune response.

A possible explanation of the contrasting effects of physiologic versus pharmacologic dosages of glucocorticoids upon resistance to respiratory infections, therefore, might be as follows: Normally the body maintains levels of hydrocortisone and immune globulins sufficient to protect against average daily exposure to infection. The lowering of resistance that follows various stresses such as excessive fatigue, lack of sleep, or emotional upset is accompanied by a relative deficiency of hydrocortisone that causes malaise and anorexia, and evidence of infection develops. When the organism is able to produce sufficient antibodies and other components of the immune response, the infection subsides and symptoms clear. The mobilization of at least some of the components of the immune response may depend upon the presence of adequate hydrocortisone, since adrenally insufficient subjects are not able to produce a normal immune response. Hence, administration of physiologic dosages of hydrocortisone (or cortisone acetate) may help to prevent the lowering of resistance that enables an infection to start or, after an infection has started, may assist the immune response and enable the organism to recover more quickly. If, however, an excessive amount of glucocorticoid is present before an infection develops, the immune response may be blocked or misdirected, allowing infections to develop and progress abnormally. It is tempting to speculate that the apparent beneficial effect of vitamin C in the common cold[27] may be mediated at least in part through the adrenals, since the highest concentration of ascorbic acid in the body occurs in the adrenal cortex.

In view of the importance of the common cold as a cause for illness and absenteeism in our economy, intensive studies of the possible protective and therapeutic effects of physiologic doses of glucocorticoids in respiratory and other infections would therefore seem desirable. It is difficult in a clinic such as ours to arrange such a study because patients do not usually report until symptoms have persisted for several days and have failed to respond to home remedies, and they often have bacterial complications by that time.

INFLUENZA

Before cortisone became available, influenza was almost invariably fatal in patients with adrenal insufficiency. As mentioned previously, therefore, when we were able to prescribe cortisone or hydrocortisone to such patients they were cautioned to increase the dosage at the onset of any infection. After it became evident that optimum maintenance therapy was between 5 mg four times daily of cortisone acetate or hydrocortisone in patients with mild adrenal insufficiency or low adrenal reserve and 10 mg four times daily for patients who had been totally adrenalectomized, such patients were routinely instructed to double the dosage of glucocorticoids at the first symptoms of onset of respiratory infection, and if they had symptoms suggestive of acute influenza, they were instructed to increase their dosage to at least 20 mg four times daily of hydrocortisone or 25 mg four times daily of cortisone acetate.

When patients followed these instructions, symptoms of fever, generalized aching, acute malaise, and anorexia often cleared within twenty-four hours, and they were able to return to work within forty-eight hours. The dosage was then gradually tapered and discontinued over the next week, and no recurrence developed, nor were there evidences of complicating bacterial infections.

The impressive improvement of these patients with steroid therapy, plus the similarity between symptoms of acute influenza and acute adrenal insufficiency, led to a decision to study plasma cortisol levels in this disease. During the epidemic of influenza in the Cleveland area in March, 1976, with the assistance of Dr. José Rivera, a primary care physician in our clinic, plasma cortisol levels were obtained on patients presenting in the acute stages of the illness. When these were found to be remarkably low, ACTH was administered to determine whether the low values were due to adrenal insufficiency. Normal responses to ACTH indicated that the adrenals were not at fault and that the defect lay in the pituitary or the hypothalamus. Furthermore, the administration of hydrocortisone, 20 mg by mouth four times daily, resulted in dramatic improvement.

Viral studies were not available in our laboratory, but Dr. Stephen Mostow agreed to study viral antibody titers on four of our patients. Two patients showed a diagnostic rise in antibody titer indicating influenza A infection; the other two had elevated titers at the time the initial blood specimen was drawn, so they could only be designated as probable acute influenza A infection. Journal editors did not consider this evidence sufficient to be acceptable for publication, possibly because of the bad reputation of glucocorticoids in infections. Further studies, therefore, must await the occurrence of another epidemic.

The results of these preliminary studies by Dr. Rivera and myself appear in Figure 7. ACTH tests in the four patients with influenza are contrasted with similar tests performed on patients with acute bacterial pharyngitis and tonsillitis.

With the technique employed, a normal unstressed subject usually has plasma cortisol levels between 18 and 32 mcg/100 ml at 8 AM and between 6 and 12 mcg/100 ml at 5 PM. The three patients with clinical influenza whose tests were performed in the morning had baseline plasma cortisol levels of only 5.8, 6.9, and 12.8 mcg, respectively, all much lower than the expected

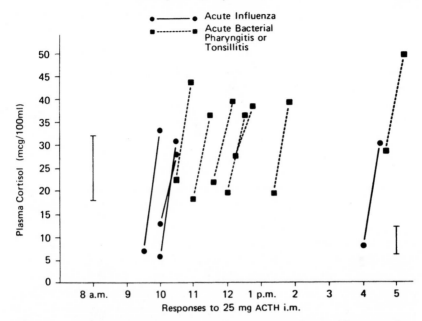

Figure 7. Plasma cortisol levels before and 30 minutes after an intramuscular injection of 25 units of cosyntropin in patients with acute influenza and in patients with acute bacterial pharyngitis or tonsillitis. The bars above 8 AM and 5 PM indicate the usual range of normal plasma cortisol levels for these times of day. Pre- and post-ACTH levels of patients are connected by lines to facilitate comparison.

normal level in the unstressed state and relatively even lower compared with the expected level during the stress of an acute infection. These tests were run on the third or fourth day of their illness, at the time they first presented themselves in the clinic for therapy.

The degree of lowering seemed to correlate with the severity of the illness, the lowest plasma cortisol occurring in the patient with the highest fever and the lowest white count and the highest plasma cortisol occurring in the patient with the lowest fever. The baseline level of the patient tested in the afternoon was in the same low range, 8.0 mcg/100 ml. Due to diurnal variation, this was within normal limits for an unstressed subject at this time of the day but low for a patient under the stress of an acute infection. The plasma cortisol levels of all four patients responded to ACTH stimulation with an increase well within normal range.

By contrast, the baseline plasma cortisol levels in all seven instances of acute bacterial pharyngitis or tonsillitis were between 18.1 and 25.5 mcg in both morning and afternoon. The plasma cortisols of these patients also responded normally to ACTH. Hence, the baseline plasma cortisol levels in patients with acute clinical influenza were impressively lower than the levels of those with acute bacterial pharyngitis or tonsillitis regardless of the time of day. The rise in plasma cortisol levels after ACTH stimulation indicated that the low baseline levels were not due to inability of the adrenals to respond. Because diurnal variation in plasma cortisol levels is known to result from the stimulation of the adrenals by endogenous ACTH, the baseline plasma cortisol levels of the patients with acute influenza were therefore similar to those that would be expected in hypopituitarism. Such findings could be due to an impaired hypothalamic-pituitary response with a decreased production of ACTH, to increased utilization of hydrocortisone associated with the infection, or to a combination of the two.

As a result of these findings, it was decided to treat patients with acute influenza in the same manner in which patients with chronic adrenal insufficiency were treated when they developed acute infections. Hydrocortisone, 20 mg by mouth four times daily before meals and at bedtime, was started. Patients were instructed to continue this dosage until they felt well, then decrease to 10 mg four times daily for two days, then 5 mg four times daily for two days, then stop. Because of initial concern regarding the possibility of complicating bacterial infection, the first three patients with influenza were also given antibiotics (erythromycin or penicillin) for seven days, but subsequent patients have received hydrocortisone without antibiotics. Supplementary multiple vitamins were also administered. Because the epidemic subsided, a total of only seven cases were treated in this manner.

Clinical responses were striking. Within twenty-four hours all patients felt much better, and within forty-eight hours symptoms such as fever, malaise, and generalized aching had completely subsided, and they felt quite well. The initial dosage of hydrocortisone was decreased after forty-eight hours and discontinued after six days of therapy. No relapses or complications occurred.

Although most fatalities occur in older patients with complicating illness that could impair resistance to any infection, at least a small percentage of deaths in influenza epidemics occur in young, apparently healthy persons,[28] suggesting an impairment of their defense response. In a pathologic report of nine cases who succumbed to influenza in the 1957 epidemic in England, all of whom were previously healthy and eight of whom were young, Roberts[29] commented on the paucity of cellular reaction in the bronchi and lungs, which were the sites of overwhelming congestion and loss of epithelium. He stated that this "apparent lack of response might be ascribed either to a depression of the tissue reaction by the virus or to overwhelming of the host by the staphylococcal infection before a tissue response could occur." He further stated that "in none of the (nine) cases was there any evidence of suprarenal damage." Because overwhelming infections characteristically cause intense stimulation of the adrenals, such pathologic findings suggest a lack of usual adrenal stimulation in response to stress.

The suggestive evidence that the impairment of response may be located at the level of the pituitary or hypothalamus has interesting implications. In view of the known effect of viruses upon formation of cellular proteins, and because both pituitary and hypothalamic hormones are protein in nature, in contrast to adrenal cortical hormones, which are steroids, it is possible that the influenza virus in some way interferes with the production of adrenocorticotropic hormone by the pituitary or of corticotropin releasing factor by the hypothalamus. Studies to answer this question, as well as the question of whether other anterior pituitary or hypothalamic hormones are affected, would, therefore, be of interest.

Why the virus appears to have more devastating effects upon some patients, even among those apparently healthy, also remains to be determined. It is evident that most patients cope with this alarming potential of the virus and recover within seven to fourteen days. Probably factors such as the virulence of the infecting agent, the size of the inoculum, and the state of resistance of the host at the time the infection develops contribute to the clinical severity.

A review of the literature revealed that in the influenza epidemic of 1958 in London, Mickerson[30] had reached similar conclusions regarding impaired pituitary response as a result of studies on four cases. At that time plasma cortisol levels were not available, but urinary excretion of 17-ketosteroids and corticoids before and after a three-day course of intramuscular corticotropin, 40 units daily, revealed that in each case urinary steroid excretion was subnormal but increased after ACTH administration. He further reported that clinical improvement occurred in all four patients after the three-day course of intramuscular ACTH. In one case no further treatment was required. In the other three cases symptoms recurred after ACTH was discontinued, so they were given prednisolone, 5 mg three times daily for one day, followed by 2.5 mg three times daily for periods ranging from two to three weeks, with uneventful recoveries. For the first five days of hospitalization each patient was given penicillin prophylactically. He also noted that in autopsy reports of patients dying with acute influenza evidence of adrenal damage was uncommon. In twenty-four necropsies of fatal influenza reported by the Public Health Laboratory Service in 1958,[31] adrenal hemorrhage was noted in only eight cases. Mickerson interpreted his observations as indicating evidence of reduced anterior pituitary activity in acute influenza.

Observations of Skanse and Miörner[32] were also interesting. In a report of the presence of preexisting untreated adrenal insufficiency in at least four and possibly five patients who succumbed to influenza in Malmö, Sweden in 1957, they noted that "resistance in Asian influenza appears to be lowered more by untreated adrenocortical insufficiency than by chronic cardiac or renal disease." They further noted that other patients with adrenal insufficiency receiving adequate substitution therapy tolerated an attack of influenza as well as, *or better than,* patients with normal adrenals. They concluded that "in all cases of severe influenza any suspected adrenal insufficiency should be compensated."

For many years it has been recognized that the clinical symptoms of acute malaise, anorexia, fever, weakness, exhaustion, and generalized aching that occur with any acute severe infection, but especially with influenza, are similar to the symptoms of acute adrenal insufficiency. It has also been known since the early days of cortisone therapy that administration of cortisone in suitable dosages to patients with acute infections such as pneumonia produced a dramatic improvement in these symptoms. The patients no longer felt ill, but the pathologic effects of the bacteria in the lungs persisted and might even progress if antibiotic therapy was not started.[1] This caused such alarm that the use of cortisone in the treatment of pneumonia was soon abandoned, even though patients receiving cortisone plus antibiotics seemed to recover nicely. The observations in our patients and in those of Mickerson strongly suggest that, in the case of influenza at least, such symptoms are actually due to inadequate adrenal response secondary to interference with hypothalamic or pituitary function. The possibility that a relative deficiency of adrenal response might be present in the incipient phase of any infectious disease should therefore be further investigated.

The evidence that the shock phase of the alarm reaction is characterized by changes consistent with relative adrenal insufficiency is consistent with this possibility, but the factors responsible for the prolongation of the shock phase in some infections are not known.

The response to treatment with physiologic dosages of hydrocortisone or cortisone in our cases in 1976 was impressive, and the absence of complications was encouraging. It is obvious that much additional experience with glucocorticoid treatment of influenza is needed before firm conclusions can be reached.

It should be borne in mind that the dosages of hydrocortisone given to these patients with influenza are dosages that are known to be helpful and even necessary to enable patients with primary adrenal insufficiency to withstand and survive acute infections such as influenza. In other words, they are physiologic dosages for patients under the stress of acute infections. Dosages much larger or much smaller than these might not be as effective and, in the case of larger dosages, might even be harmful. Similarly, if the initial dosage of 80 mg daily of hydrocortisone were continued too long, problems of hypercortisonism might develop. The principle of continuing the initial dosage until the symptoms of the illness have completely subsided, then tapering over a four-day period, has proven effective and safe so far, and it is based upon extensive previous experience in patients with primary adrenal insufficiency.

Several clinicians have reported impressive benefit from cortisone or other glucocorticoids in patients severely ill with influenza plus complicating pneumonia.[33, 34] Others have reported failure to observe convincing beneficial effects of such therapy.[35, 36] Perhaps an explanation of the discrepancy in observations may lie in the dosages or manner of administration of glucocorticoids or in the types of antibiotics administered. In none of these reports was there indication that ACTH tests or other studies of adrenal function were performed.

It should also be remembered that these cases were chosen for the study because they had uncomplicated influenza. Secondary pneumonias due to *H. influenzae,* streptococci, staphylococci, or other pathogenic bacteria are common complications of the viral infection, so if any suggestion of such complicating bacterial infections occurs, suitable antibiotic therapy in addition to the steroid therapy should be instituted promptly. It is, therefore, advisable to perform throat cultures as well as differential white blood counts and baseline plasma cortisol levels on every patient at the time of the initial visit and to perform chest x-rays on any patient who has symptoms or signs suggestive of pulmonary involvement.

If the plasma cortisol level is relatively low, supplementary hydrocortisone or cortisone acetate in dosages comparable to those used in this study may be dramatically helpful, and if there is any question regarding the possible presence of complicating bacterial infection, antibiotic therapy should be started. Patients with influenza plus a bacterial infection usually still have a relative leukopenia but with a preponderance of neutrophiles and a shift to the left in contrast to uncomplicated influenza. With such combined therapy, it is possible that the incidence of severe and fatal complications of influenza can be lessened or prevented.

Finally, these observations raise the question whether this type of response is unique for the influenza virus or whether it may occur in varying degrees with other viral illnesses. Evidence that it may occur in patients with infectious mononucleosis will be discussed. Absence of leukocytosis is characteristic, not just of influenza, but of all virus infections. This could be due at least partly to a lack of normal hydrocortisone response to stress, since hydrocortisone stimulates a granulocytic leukocytosis. The degree of lowering actually suggests a suppression of granulocytes as well. Evidence has been reported that influenza virus inhibits chemotaxis of polymorphonuclear leukocytes and monocytes,[37, 38] so this effect probably contributes to the absence of leukocytosis.

Meanwhile, it must be remembered that excessive doses of any glucocorticoid, including hydrocortisone or cortisone acetate, can impair resistance to infection as well as cause other hazardous side effects, so the indiscriminate use of these agents in infectious disease should never be undertaken.

INFECTIOUS MONONUCLEOSIS

The history of the use of physiologic dosages of glucocorticoids in infectious mononucleosis is an interesting story, demonstrating problems that have arisen as a result of the bad reputation of these agents. In 1962 Chappel[39] reported beneficial effects of cortisone therapy in 111 cases of infectious mononucleosis, including control of symptoms within a few days and elimination of long periods of bed rest and disability. Other clinicians have confirmed these beneficial effects in infectious mononucleosis with other glucocorticoids. In a study of sixty-six students with severe but uncomplicated infectious mononucleosis, Bender[40] reported that treatment with ACTH or prednisolone produced significant shortening of illness and loss of time from classes compared with matched controls. Practically all of these reports came from student health centers at universities where infectious mononucleosis is frequently encountered. Academic medical research centers, however, have been hesitant to accept these results, and medical texts recommend that glucocorticoid therapy in infectious mononucleosis be reserved for patients with more severe illness or complications. Because the clinical reports indicate that glucocorticoid therapy in dosages recommended helps to prevent such severe illness or complications, and because there has been no indication that patients with infectious mononucleosis treated with glucocorticoid therapy in the doses recommended develop any of the hazardous side effects that are so dreaded, a reconsideration of the current recommended treatment of infectious mononucleosis seems advisable.

We have also observed the impressive beneficial effects of physiological dosages of cortisone or hydrocortisone in patients with acute infectious mononucleosis. Because patients with adrenal insufficiency who develop acute infections with fever and malaise require doses of 20 mg four times daily of hydrocortisone or 25 mg four times daily of cortisone acetate, we have administered similar dosages until patients felt well, which was usually within forty-eight hours. Subsequently the dosage has been tapered to 10 mg four times daily for two days, then 5 mg four times daily for a week, before it is discontinued altogether.

After we found that plasma cortisol levels were low in acute influenza, ACTH tests were performed on patients with acute infectious mononucleosis. The results were similar to those encountered in patients with acute influenza, but the depression of plasma cortisol levels was less severe. In the initial twenty-four hours of the illness plasma cortisol levels tend to be within normal limits, but subsequently they tend to be low. Because they respond to ACTH with a normal rise it is evident that there is no impairment of adrenal cortical function, and the question again arises whether the virus is interfering with hypothalamic or pituitary response to the stress.

These observations may be related to evidence that cell-mediated immunity is impaired during acute infectious mononucleosis[41] and suggest that the effect of physiologic versus pharmacologic dosages of glucocorticoids upon cell-mediated immunity should be studied.

POST VIRAL SYNDROME

A few patients, after acute infections with influenza, infectious mononucleosis, or infectious hepatitis, have persistent symptoms of malaise, easy fatigue, and general debility lasting for several weeks to several months. After chronic fatigue from other causes was found to be frequently associated with a state of low adrenal reserve, and after patients with acute influenza or infectious mononucleosis were found to have relatively low levels of plasma cortisol, ACTH tests were run on patients with the postviral syndrome. In almost every case patients were found to have either low adrenal reserve or a low baseline plasma cortisol level, suggesting inadequate pituitary stimulation. In some patients persistently elevated viral antibody titers suggested a chronic viral infection.

When cortisone acetate or hydrocortisone, 5 mg four times daily, was given to these patients, impressive improvement in symptoms resulted. Further studies are necessary to determine why some patients develop these complications whereas others do not, but it is evident that under some circumstances viral infections can produce a persistent impairment of the pituitary-adrenal response to stress for several months and that in such cases the administration of small, physiologic dosages of cortisone acetate or hydrocortisone will produce symptomatic benefit without apparent harm.

OTHER INFECTIONS

The observations of Kass, Ingbar, and Finland[1] that cortisone can counteract the symptoms of pneumonia; of Smadel[42] and Woodward[43] and their associates that cortisone, when given in conjunction with chloramphenicol, greatly improved the clinical course of patients with typhoid fever; and of Spink[17] that glucocorticoids can improve the symptomatology and shorten the course of other severe infections all suggest that physiologic dosages of hydrocortisone or cortisone acetate might be beneficial in any severe infection, at least in its early stages. The administration of cortisone with suitable antibiotic therapy has even been reported to be helpful in tuberculosis.[44] It is apparent that in any bacterial infection glucocorticoid therapy will not replace antibiotics and, hence, glucocorticoids should be given in conjunction with appropriate antibiotics.

A number of other reports of therapeutic trials of glucocorticoids in severe infections and septic shock have appeared, and these have been summarized and criticized by Weitzman and Berger.[45] They pointed out deficiencies in adherence to standards of clinical trial design in many of these studies, including failure to follow double-blind procedure. Unfortunately, the use of double-blind procedures in studies of hormone effects is not valid unless one is studying clinical conditions where one dosage of the hormone for one duration of administration is optimum, and such conditions seldom, if ever, occur. Patients with diabetes mellitus or hypothyroidism, for example, seldom require the same dosage of insulin or thyroid medication, and assigning patients to receive glucocorticoid therapy in a single dosage for a single duration of therapy is probably no more valid than assigning patients with diabetes mellitus or hypothyroidism to receive only a single dosage of insulin or thyroid medication. If the difference between the clinical courses of steroid-treated and nontreated patients is not sufficiently great without attempts at double-blind studies, the use of steroids would not seem justified.

At any rate, further clarification of this question is needed.

REFERENCES

1. Kass EH, Ingbar SH, Finland M: Effects of adrenocorticotropic hormone in pneumonia: clinical, bacteriological and serological studies. *Ann Intern Med 33:*1081-1098, 1950.
2. Perla D, Marmorston J: *Natural Resistance and Clinical Medicine.* Boston, Little, 1941, Chap. 18, p. 475.
3. Beisel WR, Rapoport MI: Interrelations between adrenocortical functions and infectious illness. *N Engl J Med 280:*541-546, 596-604, 1969.
4. Aschoff L: *Lectures on Pathology.* New York, Hoeber, 1924, Chap. 5, p. 101.
5. Goldzieher M: *The Adrenals: Their Physiology, Pathology and Diseases.* New York, Macmillan, 1929, pp. 177-193.
6. Bosworth DC: Reversible adrenocortical insufficiency in fulminant meningococcemia. *Arch Intern Med 139:*823-824, 1979.
7. Jaffe HL, Plavska A: Functioning autoplastic suprarenal transplants. *Proc Soc Exper Biol Med 23:*528-530, 1926.
8. Marine D: Some effects of suprarenal injury on natural and acquired resistance. In *Contributions to the Medical Sciences,* in honor of Dr. E Libman by his pupils, friends and colleagues, New York, International Press, 1932.
9. Ingle DJ: Resistance of the rat to histamine shock after destruction of the adrenal medulla. Merck, *General Physiology, 118:*57, 1936.

10. Hartman FA, Scott WJM: Protection of adrenalectomized animals against bacterial intoxication by extract of adrenal cortex. *J Exp Med 55:*63-69, 1932.
11. Perla D, Marmorston-Gottesman J: Effect of injections of cortin on resistance of suprarenalectomized rats to histamine poisoning. *Proc Soc Exper Biol Med 28:*650-653, 1931.
12. Pottenger FM, Pottenger RT: Evidence of the protective influence of adrenal hormone against tuberculosis in guinea pigs. *Endocrinology 21:*529-532, 1937.
13. Whithead RW, Smith C: The effect of adrenal cortex extract on the course of certain human infections. *Proc Soc Exper Biol Med 29:*672-673, 1932.
14. Kendall EC: The adrenal cortex. *Arch Pathol 32:*474-501, 1941.
15. Benedek TG, Montgomery MM: The influence of ACTH and cortisone on the incidence of infections. *J Lab Clin Med 44:*766-767, 1954.
16. Kass EH, Finland M: Corticosteroids and infections. *Adv Intern Med 9:*45-80, 1958.
17. Spink WW: Adrenocortical steroids in the management of selected patients with infectious diseases. *Ann Intern Med 53:*1-32, 1960.
18. Ambrose CT: The essential role of corticosteroids in the induction of the immune response in vitro. In Wolstenholme GEW, Knight J (Eds.): *Hormones and the Immune Response.* Ciba Foundation Study Group No. 36, London, Churchill, 1970, pp. 100-125.
19. Pierpaoli W, Sorkin E: A thymus dependent function of the adrenal cortex and its relation to immunity. *Experientia 28:*851-852, 1972.
20. Shakelford PG, Feigin RD: Periodicity of susceptibility to pneumococcal infection: Influence of light and adrenocortical secretion. *Science 182:*285-287, 1973.
21. Jefferies, WMcK: Stimulatory effect of physiologic dosages of cortisone acetate or cortisol upon circulating levels of immunoglobulins. Unpublished paper.
22. Blanchard EW: An experimental study of opsonins in the blood. III. Further studies of their relationship to adrenocortical function. *Physiol Zoology 7:*493-508, 1934.
23. Fox C, Whitehead RW: Relation of adrenal glands to immunological processes: Effect of corticoadrenal extract on hemolysin production in normal adult laboratory animals. *J Immunol 30:*51-62, 1936.
24. White A: Influence of endocrine secretions on the structure and function of lymphoid tissue. *Harvey Lectures Ser 43:*43-70, Springfield, Thomas, 1947-48.
25. Dougherty TF, Chase JH, White A: Pituitary-adrenal cortical control of antibody release from lymphocytes. An explanation of the anamnestic response. *Proc Soc Exper Biol Med 58:*135-140, 1945.
26. Levy AL, Waldman TA: Effect of hydrocortisone on immunoglobulin metabolism. *J Clin Invest 49:*1679-1684, 1970.
27. Anderson TW, Reid DEW, Beaton GH: Vitamin C and the common cold: a double blind trial. *Can Med Assoc J 107:*503-508, 1972.

28. Oseasohn R, Adelson L, Kaji M. Clinicopathologic study of thirty-three fatal cases of Asian influenza. *N Engl J Med 260:*509-518, 1959.
29. Roberts GBS: Fulminating influenza. *Lancet ii:*944-945, 1957.
30. Mickerson JN: Influenzal pituitary depression. *Lancet i:*1110-1121, 1959.
31. Public Health Laboratory Service. *Br Med J ii:*915, 1958.
32. Skanse B, Miörner G: Asian influenza with adrenocortical insufficiency. *Lancet i:*1121-1122, 1959.
33. Plaza de los Reyes M, Cruz-Coke R, Orozco R, Matus I, Cristofafnini A: Influenzal pneumonia treated with cortisone and antibiotics. *Lancet ii:*845, 1122, 1957.
34. Rotem CE: Influenzal pneumonia treated with cortisone and antibiotics. *Lancet ii:*948, 1957.
35. Gunn W: Influenzal pneumonia treated with cortisone and antibiotics. *Lancet ii:*1004, 1957.
36. Walter WC, Douglas AC, Leckie JWH, Pines A, Grant IWB: Respiratory complications of influenza. *Lancet i:*449-454, 1958.
37. Kleinerman ES, Snyderman R, Daniels CA: Depressed monocyte chemotaxis during acute influenza infection. *Lancet ii:*1063-1066, 1975.
38. Larson HE, Blades R: Impairment of human polymorphonuclear leukocyte function by influenza virus. *Lancet i:*283, 1976.
39. Chappel MR: Infectious mononucleosis. *Southwest Med 43:*253-255, 1962.
40. Bender CE: The value of corticosteroids in the treatment of infectious mononucleosis. *JAMA 199:*529-531, 1967.
41. Mangi RJ, Niederman JC, Kelleher JE Jr, Dwyer JM, Evans AS, Kantor FS: Depression of cell-mediated immunity during acute infectious mononucleosis. *N Engl J Med 291:*1149-1153, 1974.
42. Smadel JE, Ley HL Jr., Diercks FH: Treatment of typhoid fever; combined therapy with cortisone and chloramphenicol. *Ann Intern Med 34:*1-9, 1951.
43. Woodward TE, Hall HE, Dias-Rivera R, Hightower JA, Martinez E, Parker RT: Treatment of typhoid fever: control of clinical manifestations with cortisone. *Ann Intern Med 34:*10-19, 1951.
44. Annotations: Corticosteroids for tuberculous pleural effusions. *Lancet i:*1135, 1959.
45. Weitzman S, Berger S: Clinical trial design in studies of corticosteroids in bacterial infections. *Ann Intern Med 81:*36-42, 1974.

Chapter 10

MISCELLANEOUS CLINICAL CONDITIONS IN WHICH THERE APPEARS TO BE A PROMISING THERAPEUTIC POTENTIAL FOR PHYSIOLOGIC DOSAGES OF GLUCOCORTICOIDS

IN CHAPTERS 4, 5, 6, 7, and 8 clinical uses of physiologic dosages of hydrocortisone and cortisone acetate in conditions in which their use has been either established or indicated for logical reasons have been discussed. I would now like to discuss other conditions in which, for various reasons, therapeutic promise also seems likely. In some of these conditions, the rationale for their use is also logical, but in others, at first glance their use would seem contraindicated, at least on the basis of popular understanding of their actions.

HIRSUTISM

Although racial and familial factors contribute to the sensitivity of hair follicles to stimulation, the source of stimulation of coarse hair growth on the face or body is androgen. This is produced normally by the adrenals and testes and under certain abnormal circumstances by the ovaries. In addition, other tissues may be capable of converting precursors to androgens.

In a recent study of fourteen patients with hirsutism, Gibson and his associates[1] found evidence of abnormality of adrenal response to ACTH in all except three. In five patients evidence suggested a partial deficiency of 3β-hydroxysteroid dehydrogenase Δ 4-5 isomerase and in five others a partial deficiency of 11β-hydroxylase. Also, in six patients an abnormally high increment of dehydroepiandrosterone relative to hydrocortisone was noted. Hence, patients with hirsutism as well as those with ovarian dysfunction have a high incidence of abnormal adrenal steroid metabolism.

Androgen excess causes increased hair growth on the beard

area, trunk, and extremities and a thinning of scalp hair. Evidence of excessive androgen production is manifested by increased urinary excretion of 17-KS or by elevated plasma levels of testosterone or of DHA sulfate.

Women with complaints of hirsutism or thinning of scalp hair will often be helped by the administration of small, subreplacement dosages of hydrocortisone, suggesting that the hirsutism and/or thinning of scalp hair results from a pathologic process similar to that which causes congenital adrenal hyperplasia, or by some autoimmune disorder. In some cases, plasma ACTH may be elevated prior to treatment. Improvement is slow in becoming evident, however, apparently due to the property of hair follicles that causes them, once they have produced coarse hairs, to continue to grow coarse hairs until they are replaced by fine ones. Because hairs are replaced at intervals of up to eighteen months, a patient may have to continue treatment for a year or more before appreciable improvement is noted. Also, unless the dosage of hydrocortisone is increased during periods of stress, the production of androgen at those times of increased adrenal activity may be sufficient to maintain the hirsutism. Furthermore, the excessive production of androgen must be suppressed throughout the twenty-four-hour period, and this is difficult with the short-acting preparations available today. The advantage of a four-times-daily schedule versus a two-times-daily schedule in reducing elevated androgen production is demonstrated in Figure 4.

When treatment is continued regularly for eighteen months or longer, most patients will note some diminution of excessive hair growth and some return of thinned scalp hair, but beneficial effects are seldom dramatic. It is my impression that patients who have received the greatest benefit have been those who have followed instructions regarding therapy most carefully. It is difficult for many patients to appreciate the necessity of taking medication regularly, especially for a condition as benign as hirsutism, so they often forget doses or fail to increase doses during infections or other acute stresses.

Some patients appear to have excess androgen from the ovaries or from both the ovaries and adrenals.[2-4] In such cases the pathologic physiology appears to involve a relative deficiency of an enzyme in the pathway of production of estrogen that results in an excessive production of androgenic precursors, and an elevated level of follicle-stimulating hormone (FSH) in the blood or urine may be helpful in indicating their source. The administration of small, physiologic doses of estrogens, such as 0.3 mg estrone sulfate daily except during menses, will help in correcting the disorder, but again it is necessary to continue treatment for a year or longer before improvement becomes manifest. In patients with disorders of both the adrenals and ovaries, such as the Stein-Leventhal syndrome,[5] both hydrocortisone and estrogen must be given simultaneously. If the woman needs estrogen, it will not interfere with the regularity of her menstrual cycles; on the contrary, it will make them more normal, in contrast to women who do not need estrogen, whose ovulations may be delayed and cycles prolonged by such estrogen administration.

Recently there has been concern expressed regarding the safety of estrogen therapy due to statistical evidence that women given estrogens at the menopause had a higher incidence of endometrial cancer than those who received no estrogen. It was feared that the estrogen therapy might have in some way contributed to the development of cancer.

It is unlikely that physiologic dosages of a normal hormone would cause cancer. If they did, the highest incidence of cancer of the endometrium would be in young women because they have the highest physiologic levels of estrogen. It is not surprising that estrogen administration at the menopause is associated with a statistically higher incidence of carcinoma of the uterus or breast, because these tissues are dependent upon estrogen for their normal development, but in such cases estrogen would merely be a permissive factor, not a causative factor. It is unfortunate that this distinction has not been publicized, because many women with estrogen deficiency, especially young women, are being frightened from taking a hormone that they need for normal development and health. Synthetic estrogens such as diethylstilbestrol, on the other hand, introduce proven potential hazards, so they are contraindicated at any time.

In my experience with administration of physiologic dosages of normal estrogens such as conjugated estrogens, ethinyl estradiol, and 17-beta-estradiol, no untoward effects have been encountered. They are routinely administered on a cyclic schedule. Replacement dosages are taken for three weeks, then omitted for a week. Subreplacement dosages, on the other hand, are usually prescribed to promote more normal ovulatory cycles, so they are taken until menses start, then omitted until menses stop. The nausea that has been reported with estrogen therapy apparently results from larger doses, as patients treated as described have not complained of nausea.

There is evidence that androgen can be produced from precursor steroids in peripheral tissues, and this is thought to cause hirsutism in some cases. If it does, it must be either under ACTH or FSH control or a manifestation of an autoimmune process, because in every case of hirsutism I have been able to study, the excessive levels of androgen in blood or urine or the hirsutism itself have improved with administration of hydrocortisone or cortisone acetate or estrogen or a combination of one of the former with the latter.

Case 1 is that of a woman who presented with a problem of hirsutism and who has been followed for thirty years.

Case 1

The patient was referred in 1950 at the age of twenty-two because of increased hair growth on her chin, which had been noted for about a year. For several months she used a depilatory, but it seemed to be getting worse, so she consulted a dermatologist, who started electrolysis. Her health had otherwise been good. The menarche had occurred at age twelve and cycles had been regular, with intervals of thirty days, menses lasting four days. Family history was negative for endocrine disorder. Physical examination was normal except for slight increase in hair growth on the chin, periareolar and subumbilical areas, and mild acne of the chin. The clitoris was not enlarged. Urinary 17-KS were in the high normal range. The patient was assured that there was no evidence of endocrine tumor, but no other treatment was known at the time.

She returned five years later with evidence of progression of hair growth to include moderately severe hirsutism of the face, chest, periareolar and subumbilical areas, and legs. She also had moderate acne of the chin and shoulders. During the previous six months she had missed one menstrual period, and another had occurred after an interval of six weeks. Breast development was at the lower limit of normal. Urinary 17-KS were 24.6 mg/24 hours, and a repeat determination was 24.0 mg/24 hours.

Because of the slow progression, it was thought likely that she had a functional disorder of adrenal steroid metabolism, so she was given hydrocortisone, 5 mg every eight hours. A month later urinary 17-KS were 11.0 mg/24 hours, consistent with the impression that this was a case of functional steroid disorder rather than a tumor. Six months later there was definite evidence of decrease in hair growth with softening of the texture of the hairs. The dosage of hydrocortisone was increased to 5 mg four times daily, and this resulted in a decrease in urinary 17-KS to 7.5 mg/24 hours. She continued to take hydrocortisone, 5 mg four times daily, until 1967, when cortisone acetate, 5 mg four times daily, was substituted. In 1970 the dosage was decreased to 2.5 mg four times daily for eighteen months, but she developed eczema, so the dosage was returned to 5 mg four times daily. This has been continued up to the present, the eczema having subsided except for occasional mild occurrences.

During her treatment the patient has married and had three full-term pregnancies. Excessive hair gradually improved so that she had to pluck only an occasional coarse hair from her chin, and her complexion remained clear. In 1975, after the patient had taken physiologic dosages of hydrocortisone or cortisone acetate for eighteen years, an ACTH test showed a baseline plasma cortisol of 15μg% at 12 noon and an increase to 27.9 μg% thirty minutes after an I.M. injection of 25 units of Cortrosyn. Plasma testosterone while taking cortisone acetate, 5 mg four times daily, was 25 ng/dl, well within normal range.

This case demonstrates not only the effectiveness of small doses of cortisone and hydrocortisone in hirsutism and acne but also its safety over an extended period of administration.

A second patient was referred primarily for excessive hair growth, but she also had acne and irregular menses.

Case 2

This young woman was referred at the age of twenty-two years. She had noted some dark hair on her face and body in childhood, but this had become progressively worse since the menarche at age fifteen. Her cycles had been irregular, with intervals of two to eight weeks, menses lasting four to five days with clots and cramps on the first day. Her gynecologist had given her an oral contraceptive for three months, and subsequently her cycles had been slightly more regular, but they still varied with intervals from two to five weeks. She also suffered from moderate acne, worse premenstrually. She had had eczema since infancy, with allergy tests and injections between ages five and nine years. A "cortisone" ointment had been beneficial.

Physical examination revealed a well-developed and nourished young woman with moderately severe hirsutism of the face, neck, periareolar and subumbilical areas, sternum, and extremities. There was moderate acne of the shoulders and back, mild of the face. The thyroid was not enlarged. Mild chronic cystic mastitis was present. The remainder of her examination was within normal limits. Urinary 17-KS were 10.2 mg/24 hours.

On Cortef, 5 mg four times daily, her complexion cleared completely, and hair growth on the face diminished impressively. Plasma testosterone remained elevated, however, measuring 202 ng/dl with an upper limit of normal of 80 ng/dl for a female. The dosage of hydrocortisone was therefore increased to 7.5 mg four times daily, and plasma testosterone decreased to 44 ng/dl. On this therapy not only did the complexion remain clear and hair growth diminish, especially on her face, but menstrual cycles also became regular, and her basal temperature chart showed evidence of ovulation about the fourteenth day of twenty-eight to thirty day cycles. Clotting and severe cramps with her menses disappeared, cystic mastitis cleared, and her eczema remained in remission. After two years the dosage of hydrocortisone was reduced to 5 mg four times daily. Plasma testosterone remained within normal range and clinical improvement persisted, so this dosage has been continued for an additional three years.

This young woman, who had been referred primarily for hirsutism, experienced marked improvement not only in this problem but also in acne, chronic cystic mastitis, irregular menses, dysmenorrhea, and eczema, suggesting that all of these disorders had some common factor in their etiology.

ACNE

Acne can be caused by excessive production of androgen in men and women, but it may result from other factors such as ingestion of iodide or chocolate, or skin irritation by certain oils encountered in industry or in cosmetics and hair sprays. If the latter are ruled out, the administration of small physiologic doses of hydrocortisone or cortisone acetate may produce dramatic improvement. In women, the combination of small doses of hydrocortisone and small doses of estrogen may be necessary for patients who have excess androgen from both adrenals and ovaries, and occasionally patients are encountered whose acne results from excess androgen from the ovaries only and who will improve with estrogen therapy alone. The latter usually have associated ovarian dysfunction and slightly high FSH levels. Those whose acne results from adrenal dysfunction may or may not have associated ovarian dysfunction; this apparently depends upon whether the adrenal dysfunction includes an excessive production of estrogen by the adrenals. A characteristic of acne due to adrenal androgen is accentuation with or after stress and before and during menses. The former is undoubtedly due to the increased adrenocortical stimulation that occurs with stress. The latter probably also results from increased adrenocortical stimulation associated with the production of adrenal estrogen at this time of the menstrual cycle. An elevation of urinary 17-KS or of plasma testosterone or DHA sulfate levels is found in patients with acne due to adrenal or ovarian dysfunction, and the latter is usually associated with slight elevation of plasma FSH. The former may or may not be associated with slight elevation of plasma ACTH. Improvement in acne is manifest much sooner than in hirsutism and should be evident within a month when therapy is effective. An exception is cystic acne such as that described in Case 3 following, where an autoimmune factor may be involved and improvement is slower.

The beneficial effect of small doses of glucocorticoids in acne is so impressive and so safe that it warrants much wider use. Dermatologists have naturally been hesitant to use larger dosages of glucocorticoids that might produce harmful side effects in such a benign clinical condition, but the administration of 5 mg of hydrocortisone four times daily is not only more physiologic but also as safe as, or safer than, the use of broad spectrum antibiotics that is popular in the treatment of acne today. Even the more severe cystic forms of acne may respond dramatically to this type of physiologic therapy, but improvement in cystic acne tends to be much slower, sometimes requiring several months before becoming apparent. Beneficial results in acne are not confined to females, for males with this skin disorder seem to respond equally well.

Case 3 is an example of severe cystic acne that cleared while the patient was receiving low dosage glucocorticoid therapy.

Case 3
This young woman was referred at the age of twenty-seven because of

cystic acne that had started six months previously in the sixth month of her first pregnancy. The menarche had occurred at age twelve, and cycles had been regular with intervals of twenty-eight to thirty days, menses lasting five to six days. She had been married for three years and had used an oral contraceptive for two years, conceiving six months after discontinuing it. Her pregnancy was uneventful until the sixth month, when she developed progressive severe cystic acne. This persisted after a full-term, normal delivery. After having no resumption of spontaneous menses by eight weeks post partum, she was given medication that caused withdrawal flow. In addition, tetracycline, three times daily for two months, had been given for the acne without benefit. She was then advised to resume the oral contraceptive, and three weeks after resuming this, when there was still no evidence of improvement of the acne, she was referred to me. Her health had otherwise been good. She had been adopted in infancy, and her family history was not known.

Physical examination revealed severe cystic acne of the face, neck, chest, and back, rather poor breast development, and a functional systolic murmur over the precordium. The clitoris was not enlarged, and there was no hirsutism. Urinary 17-KS were 6.1 mg/24 hrs, and plasma testosterone was less than 30 ng/dl.

Although there was no laboratory evidence of hormonal abnormality, the onset of acne during her pregnancy suggested the possibility of a hormonal relationship; the beneficial effects of physiologic dosages of hydrocortisone in other types of acne, as well as their safety, resulted in a decision to try this type of therapy. Cortef, 5 mg four times daily, was therefore prescribed. Over the next six months there was gradual but progressive improvement. The addition of Premarin, 0.3 mg twice daily except during menses for six months, did not produce significant additional benefit, so it was discontinued. An increase in hydrocortisone to 7.5 mg four times daily seemed to cause further improvement, so this was continued. Her acne cleared completely, and regular, ovulatory menstrual cycles resumed.

The preceding patient therefore had a clearing of severe cystic acne on physiologic doses of hydrocortisone, even though hormone studies gave no evidence of abnormality prior to therapy. The development of acne during her pregnancy, with slower response to glucocorticoid therapy, suggests a different cause from the more common type of acne. Perhaps her cystic acne may have been related to an autoimmune factor.

An example of a male with cystic acne who improved on low dosage glucocorticoid therapy at the same time he was being treated for infertility is presented in case 4.

Case 4

This young man was seen in consultation at the age of twenty-four years because of infertility and low semen volume with low motility (volume 0.5 ml., 60.06 million/ml, 40% motile). He had had cystic acne of his face and chest for approximately eight years, had been married for three years, and tried unsuccessfully for a pregnancy for the previous year. Urinary 17-KS were 16.3 mg/24 hours, and plasma estrogen was 128 pg/ml with the upper limit of normal for a male 70 pg/ml. Plasma cortisol at 9 AM was 16.2 mcg%; thirty minutes after an I.M. injection of 25 units of Cortrosyn this rose to 35.0 mcg%. On Cortef, 5 mg four times daily, sperm count increased to 105 million per cc, but volume remained low. His cystic acne cleared completely, but his wife did not conceive until he had a varicocele corrected by surgery. Subsequently his wife had a normal baby.

The relatively rapid clearing of this man's acne is more characteristic of the response of this disorder to small doses of cortisone acetate or hydrocortisone, and the safety of this therapy has resulted in the patient continuing it after his fertility problem had been corrected.

CHRONIC CYSTIC MASTITIS

The presence of diffuse induration of the glandular tissue of the breasts, sometimes accompanied by cystic nodules, may occur with irregular menses or with apparently normal cycles. The condition is usually most pronounced premenstrually, and it has been attributed to a relative deficiency of progesterone relative to estrogen, since some cases may be helped by the administration of small doses of progesterone during the luteal phase. When low dosage glucocorticoid therapy has been administered for ovarian dysfunction, associated cystic mastitis has diminished or cleared in practically every case. We have, therefore, tried this therapy in patients with cystic mastitis without apparent ovarian dysfunction, and it has been equally effective. Presumably the mild disorder of steroid metabolism that is responsible for this condition is benefited by small doses of glucocorticoid.

DYSMENORRHEA

It has been estimated that 30 to 50 percent of women of childbearing age suffer from excessively painful menstrual cramps, often associated with nausea, vomiting, diarrhea, headache, fatigue, and nervousness. It has recently been demonstrated that most of these women have an excessive concentration of prostaglandins E and F_{2a} in their menstrual fluid, often two to three times higher on the first day or two of menstruation than in women who have no dysmenorrhea, and administration of prostaglandin inhibitors, such as ibuprofen, indomethacin, mefenamic acid, and naproxen-sodium, often provides symptomatic relief.[6] Women with ovarian dysfunction often have dysmenorrhea, and when their ovarian dysfunction has benefited from subreplacement dosages of cortisone acetate or hydrocortisone, dysmenorrhea has also disappeared. Hence, such therapy might be helpful in patients with dysmenorrhea with regular menses. It would also be advisable to determine the effect of small doses of glucocorticoids upon prostaglandin content of the menstrual fluid.

HYPOTHYROIDISM WITH HIGH CIRCULATING T_3

In 1967 Refetoff, DeWind, and DeGroot[7] reported a familial syndrome that included some symptoms and signs of hypothyroidism associated with an elevated level of serum protein-bound iodine (PBI). Subsequent studies revealed that the high PBI was due to elevated levels of circulating thyroxine (T_4) and triiodothyronine (T_3)[8] that could result from a defect at the level of nuclear receptors.[9] Other reports of patients with apparent partial peripheral resistance to thyroid hormone have appeared subsequently,[10-15] with considerable variability in clinical features.

In 1950 Hill, Reiss, Forsham, and Thorn,[16] in their studies of the effects of ACTH or cortisone in patients with thyroid disorders, reported that administration of either ACTH or cortisone acetate appeared to be capable of increasing basal metabolic rate without changing the level of serum protein-bound iodine of patients taking a constant dose of thyroid. In this same year Beierwaltes and his associates[17] reported that cortisone seemed to have a calorigenic effect in two patients with untreated myxedema. The following year Werner and his associates[18] reported evidence that cortisone administration to a patient with myxedema resulted in an increase in BMR, serum protein-bound iodine, and I^{131} uptake and a decrease in serum cholesterol. In 1952 Lerman, Harington, and Means,[19] in a report of physiologic activity of some analogues of thyroxine, described a patient with myxedema who responded poorly to intravenous thyroxine until "cortisone in a dosage of 50 mg twice a day was added." Then "metabolism rose speedily to normal values." The authors then commented that "this type of response ... may have an important bearing on the fundamental mechanism of the action of thyroid hormone on the cell." Commenting on these studies in 1953, Thorn and his associates[20] stated, "The interesting possibility arises that cortisone aids in the peripheral utilization of thyroid hormone."

Three years ago a patient was seen in consultation who had some symptoms of hypothyroidism associated with an elevated level of circulating T_3, and her symptoms and laboratory findings were restored to normal by cortisone acetate in a dosage of 5 mg 4 times daily.

Case 5

A fifty-five year old female was referred in 1977 because of chronic fatigue for six years. She had an operation for a strangulated hernia at age forty and subsequently began to tire easily. Six years prior to referral fatigue became worse and she saw a physician who made a diagnosis of possible collagen disorder. Latex fixation and lupus erythematosus tests had been negative. A five-hour glucose tolerance test had been normal except for a slightly low blood sugar level (68 mg%) at the third hour. A neurologist had been consulted, and a diagnosis of Raynaud's phenomenon and possible chronic depression was made. Skull x-rays and an electroencephalogram were normal. She had been given amitriptyline HCL (Elavil®) briefly without benefit. She drank up to ten cups of coffee daily in an attempt to obtain energy, but fatigue persisted, so she was referred for endocrine evaluation. She had four children, had experienced an apparently normal menopause at age forty-nine, about the time symptoms of fatigue increased, and she had received no estrogen therapy. She was sensitive to cold; her hair tended to be dry, but bowels had been regular. A sister had a goiter, but family history was otherwise negative for endocrine disorder.

Physical examination revealed a moderately overweight female with a height of 61¼ inches, weight 156 lbs., blood pressure 124/70, pulse 96 and regular. Her skin was quite dry, and her voice was low-pitched and slightly hoarse. The thyroid gland was not palpable. Reflexes were equal and within normal limits. The remainder of her examination was within normal limits. Hemoglobin was 13.8 gm, WBC .7,840, with 63 percent neutrophils, 28 percent lymphocytes, 6 percent monocytes, 1 percent eosinophils, and 2 percent basophils. T_3 sponge uptake was 29 percent, T_4 was 9.2 μg/dl, and T_3 by RIA was 250 ng/dl. Plasma cortisol at 3 PM was 23.5 μg/dl; thirty minutes after 25 units of Cortrosyn I.M. this rose to 40.5 μg/dl. Total proteins were 6.7 gm/dl, with 4.5 gm albumin and 2.2 gm globulin.

She was told to stop drinking coffee. This improved her ability to sleep; her resting pulse rate decreased to 76 per minute, but chronic fatigue persisted. Because of the evidence for impairment of utilization of T_3, plus the observation that a number of patients given small dosages of cortisone acetate or hydrocortisone for other problems had experienced an improvement in energy on this medication, a trial with this treatment was suggested. After discussion she agreed to such a trial, so cortisone acetate, 5 mg by mouth four times daily, was started.

When she returned two months later, she reported that she had begun to feel dramatically better about two days after starting the medication, that her energy was now fine, that she no longer had insomnia but fell asleep as soon as her head hit the pillow, and she had resumed playing golf twice weekly. Improvement was so impressive that she went to the library and read more about her adrenals and cortisone, and this made her worried. She tried stopping the cortisone but became chronically fatigued again, so she resumed it and her energy returned. Her husband was so impressed with her improvement that he reminded her to take the medication regularly. While taking the cortisone her T_3 sponge uptake was 45 percent, T_4 was 9.8 μg/dl, and T_3 by RIA was 135 ng/dl. Plasma cortisol at 11 AM was 23 μg/dl and after Cortrosyn rose to 39 ug/dl.

The patient has subsequently taken cortisone for three years and has continued to feel well. She tried stopping it again but developed chronic fatigue after about a week, so it was resumed. She stated, "I just cannot believe this medication could make such a tremendous difference in the way I feel, both mentally and physically."

Subsequently two similar cases with variable symptoms of hypothyroidism and elevated blood levels of T_3 by RIA have been encountered, and these have improved with treatment with hydrocortisone, 5 mg four times daily, even though ACTH tests were within the lower range of normal. It therefore appears that small doses of cortisone acetate or hydrocortisone can correct a partial receptor block for T_3, and it would be interesting to determine whether this therapy would benefit the more severe degrees of block that have been reported previously.

Further studies in other patients[21] have demonstrated that treatment with small dosages of cortisone acetate or hydrocortisone is associated with a decrease in circulating T_3 by RIA when initial levels are high normal or elevated, suggesting that these physiologic dosages improve peripheral utilization of thyroid hormone (Fig. 8). In patients whose initial levels of T_3 by RIA were low normal or low, treatment with these dosages was associated with an increase in T_3 by RIA while patients reported improvement in energy, suggesting that they increased conversion of T_4 to T_3, another mechanism by which they might improve peripheral utilization of thyroid hormone. This would contrast with the effect of larger dosages of glucocorticoids, which appear to decrease the conversion of T_4 to T_3.[22]

If these observations can be confirmed, the predictions of Lerman, Harington, and Means[19] and of Thorn and his group[20] will have been fulfilled. At any rate, patients with symptoms of hypothyroidism associated with high circulating T_3 by RIA and those with evidence of a block in conversion of T_4 to T_3 warrant

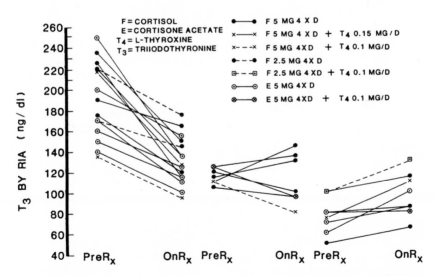

Figure 8. Effect of physiologic dosages of cortisone acetate (E) or cortisol (F) on circulating T_3. Left: — subjects whose baseline T_3 was 130 ng/dl or higher; center — subjects whose baseline T_3 was 105-125; right — subjects whose baseline T_3 was 100 or less.

therapeutic trials with small dosages of cortisone acetate or hydrocortisone. Patients with a number of acute and chronic nonthyroidal illnesses as well as those with starvation have often been found to have low serum T_3 and normal serum T_4 levels,[23] suggesting either an increased utilization of T_3 or a physiologic decrease in conversion of T_4 to T_3, so these must be differentiated from those with a pathologic decrease in conversion of T_4 to T_3.

FUNCTIONAL HYPOGLYCEMIA

In recent years the lay press has emphasized the importance of functional hypoglycemia as a cause of unexplained symptoms, especially chronic fatigue, in many persons. The occurrence of an abnormally low blood sugar after a test dose of glucose implies either an abnormally large production of insulin in response to the glucose or a decreased ability of the body to protect against hypoglycemia. Because hydrocortisone appears to be the body's chief defense against abnormally low blood sugar levels, we have routinely run ACTH tests on patients who are referred with a diagnosis of functional hypoglycemia. In almost every case we have encountered to date, low adrenal reserve has been demonstrated. It is not surprising that functional hypoglycemia should be a manifestation of low adrenal reserve, but this has not been emphasized in the literature. In such cases, the administration of small physiologic dosages of cortisone acetate or hydrocortisone has produced impressive, and sometimes dramatic, improvement. Two case summaries will exemplify the value of this type of therapy.

Case 6

This fifty-two year old male was referred because of hypoglycemia. His first symptom had been a transient dizzy spell while at lunch with business associates. He had drunk several cups of coffee that morning, so he stopped drinking coffee, but occasional spells of increased nervousness, palpitations, and weakness continued especially in the morning or evening. A five-hour glucose tolerance test at another clinic had shown relatively low blood sugars at the third, fourth, and fifth hours. Valium had been prescribed as symptomatic therapy. He had been under considerable tension during the previous year and had experienced more fatigue. Vitiligo had been present, gradually progressive over the previous five years. His father had senile diabetes and hypertension, and one sister had a diagnosis of low blood sugar and allergies.

Physical examination revealed a height of 72¼ inches, weight 189½ pounds, blood pressure 140/95, pulse 60 and regular. There was moderate vitiligo of the hands, arms, and chest. The thyroid was not palpable, and there was no lymphadenopathy. The liver edge was palpable one finger-breadth below the right costal margin, not tender. The remainder of his examination was within normal limits. An SMA-12 was normal. T_3 sponge uptake was 58 percent, and T_4 was 6.6 mcg%. Plasma cortisol at 8 AM was 18.3, and post-ACTH this rose to 27.0 μg%.

Because of the evidence of low adrenal reserve with functional hypoglycemia, he was given a prescription for Cortef, 5 mg four times daily. On this medication impressive improvement occurred; energy returned to normal, and symptoms of hypoglycemia did not recur. An ACTH test a year later revealed a plasma cortisol at 10:45 AM of 14.1 mcg; 30 minutes after Cortrosyn this rose to 21.4 μg%. Cortef was therefore continued. Two years subsequently a repeat ACTH test showed a baseline plasma cortisol of 14 at 10 AM; thirty minutes after ACTH this rose to 22 μg%. He has continued to take Cortef, 5 mg three times daily, and has continued to feel well.

At the time of his last visit, three and one-half years after beginning therapy, weight was 194¼ pounds with shoes, blood pressure 114/70, pulse 80 with occasional premature beats. He has stopped drinking caffeine-containing beverages, but he continues to smoke up to one pack of cigarettes daily. The liver edge is still palpable one finger-breadth below the right costal margin. An SMAC was normal, including normal cholesterol, triglycerides, alkaline phosphatase, bilirubin, LDH and SGOT.

Case 7

The patient was referred at the age of twenty-three years because of functional hypoglycemia. He had been having intermittent symptoms of weakness, palpitation, and anxiety for nine months with onset shortly after an attack of "intestinal flu." He had been referred to a neurologist a month previously, but neurologic examination and electroencephalogram were within normal limits. His general health had been good, and he had had no serious illnesses or operations. A five-hour glucose tolerance test had shown hypoglycemia at three hours.

Physical examination was within normal limits except for mild acne and a positive Chvostek's sign. Height was 70¼ inches, weight 169½ pounds, blood pressure 100/70, pulse 120 and regular. An SMAC was normal. Plasma cortisol at 8:30 AM was 18.5μg%; thirty minutes after Cortrosyn this rose to 27.4μg%.

A diagnosis of low adrenal reserve and hyperventilation syndrome was made, and he was given cortisone acetate, 5 mg four times daily. On this program his symptoms of weakness and palpitation cleared and energy returned impressively. He also experienced improvement in

acne, for which he had been treated by a dermatologist with variable
results. A repeat ACTH test later showed a plasma cortisol at 12 noon of
11.5 mcg%; thirty minutes after Cortrosyn this rose to 20 mcg%. He has
continued to take Cortef, 5 mg four times daily, chiefly because of its
benefit to his complexion, and he has continued to feel well.

Johnson and her associates[24] have recently pointed out the
lack of correlation between the level of plasma glucose nadir,
rate of glucose descent after reaching its peak, presence of
hypoglycemic symptoms, and increase in cortisol level in patients suspected of having reactive hypoglycemia, so it would be
interesting to determine whether ACTH tests would be helpful.
Based on our experience, they should be.

UNEXPLAINED CHRONIC FATIGUE

Every practicing physician has encountered a number of patients complaining of unexplained chronic fatigue. When a
routine history and physical examination plus urinalysis, blood
counts, and screening blood chemistries fail to reveal any abnormalities, many of these patients have been referred to psychia-
trists, who usually find no significant psychiatric disorder. These
patients differ from neurotics in that they seem to be anxious to
be active and work, but they feel too tired to undertake or
accomplish the things they would like to do. Conditions that
should be ruled out include mild hypothyroidism, low-grade
chronic infection of a tooth, of the sinuses, or of the urinary tract
that has been otherwise asymptomatic, or obscure malignancy.

If none of these conditions are found, an ACTH test should be
performed, as many of these patients will be found to have low
adrenal reserve or a low baseline plasma cortisol level, suggesting inadequate stimulation of the adrenal by the pituitary. These
findings are characteristic of the postviral fatigue syndrome, as
discussed in Chapter 9, but they also may occur in chronic
allergies as discussed in Chapter 7. In such cases impressive
symptomatic improvement will occur with administration of 5
mg cortisone acetate or hydrocortisone four times daily. Most
allergies, in addition to causing fatigue, have characteristic manifestations of urticaria, dermatitis, rhinitis, asthma, gastrointestinal disorders, or headaches, but sometimes fatigue seems to be
the only symptom.

Occasionally a patient is encountered complaining of chronic fatigue whose ACTH test is normal, and no other evidence of abnormality can be found. Psychoneurosis or depression seems unlikely because characteristic symptoms are absent and patients with depression usually have an excessive adrenal response to ACTH stimulation,[25, 26] yet a therapeutic trial with small doses of cortisone acetate or hydrocortisone may produce symptomatic benefit. This effect came as a surprise, and I was inclined to attribute it to the presence of an undetected mild allergy until recently when it was noted that the administration of these dosages of cortisone acetate or hydrocortisone can result in a decrease in circulating T_3 by RIA. Early in this chapter a patient was described with symptoms of hypothyroidism and a high T_3 by RIA, suggesting a partial receptor block for triiodothyronine that was corrected by cortisone acetate, 5 mg four times daily. It was also noted that when patients with baseline T_3 by RIA levels in the high normal range were given small dosages of cortisone acetate or hydrocortisone for any reason, such as irregular menses or hirsutism, the T_3 by RIA level decreased at the time the patient reported an improvement in energy. The possibility must therefore be considered that at least part of the clinical improvement associated with administration of small doses of these steroids may result from an increased uptake of triiodothyronine by the cells. This observation also suggests that a basic mechanism of action of physiologic dosages of glucocorticoids may be an increased cellular uptake of triiodothyronine. This possibility, as well as the possibility that utilization of other hormones or metabolic substances might be enhanced in this fashion, should be investigated further, since this might be a mechanism of the "permissive effect" of glucocorticoids suggested by Ingle[27] or of their effect as biological amplifiers.[28]

TRAVEL FATIGUE (JET LAG)

In Chapter 3 it was noted that a diurnal variation in plasma cortisol levels occurs normally, with a peak shortly after arising following a good night's sleep and a low point shortly after retiring at night. When a person travels to different time zones, especially when differences of several hours occur, adjustment of the hypothalamic-pituitary-adrenal axis to the new sleep-wake schedule may require five to ten days. Meanwhile, the person tends to feel chronically fatigued. Because patients on low dosage glucocorticoid therapy do not seem to experience this "jet lag," presumably because their therapeutic program tends to decrease diurnal variation and because they adjust their dosage schedule to the new time schedule immediately, a short course of 5 mg cortisone acetate or hydrocortisone four times daily may be an effective yet safe method of avoiding or treating this disorder.

LEUKEMIA AND LYMPHOMA

The reports that glucocorticoid therapy produces lysis of lymphoid tissue resulted in therapeutic trials with pharmacological dosages in patients with lymphoid leukemia and lymphoma. Although transient beneficial effects were observed in patients with both acute and chronic lymphoid leukemia and in patients with lymphoma, there was no apparent effect on the ultimate outcome of these diseases. Relatively short courses of pharmacologic dosages of glucocorticoids are still being used in conjunction with combined therapy with chemotherapeutic and cytotoxic agents in these disorders. In view of the safety of prolonged uses of physiologic dosages and because, they seem to enhance immunity, a property that seems to be important in resistance to malignancy as well as to infections, the prolonged administration of physiologic dosages of cortisone or hydrocortisone, alone or in conjunction with chemotherapeutic or cytotoxic agents in such disorders, seems worth studying.

CARCINOMA OF THE BREAST OR THE PROSTATE

Two other types of malignancy in which therapy directed towards the adrenal gland has shown evidence of at least temporary benefit have been carcinomas of the breast and of the prostate gland. Since normal breast development depends upon adequate estrogen stimulation, it was not surprising to find that many cases of cancer of the breast seem to be partly dependent upon estrogen stimulation. In such cases, removal of the ovaries, the major source of estrogen in premenopausal women, has produced impressive benefit, although this has been only temporary. After cortisone acetate and hydrocortisone became available, it became surgically feasible to remove the adrenal glands, the other glandular source of estrogen, and in such patients further clinical remissions, sometimes of several years duration, occurred. Ultimately, the cancer would begin to grow again, however, so such procedures were still of only temporary benefit.

Because total adrenalectomy is a major surgical procedure that is not available in all hospitals, attempts were made to suppress the adrenal production of estrogen by the administration of suitable dosages of glucocorticoids, and in such cases, temporary remissions have also been observed. A suppressive dosage of 10 mg four times daily of hydrocortisone in the unstressed state will inhibit the adrenal production of estrogen. This also tends to make the patients' adrenals sluggish so that they will not react to stress in an adequate fashion, so such patients must be given additional steroid at times of stress as though they were adrenally insufficient. As long as the basic dosage of hydrocortisone does not exceed 10 mg four times daily, they will not develop evidence of hypercortisonism, however. Physiologic dosages of androgen will help to protect against the easy bruisability and ecchymoses that accompany deficiency of adrenal androgen.

With recent evidence that the presence of estrogen receptors in malignant tissue may determine the effectiveness of ablative therapy directed towards the ovaries or adrenals or both, there has been emphasis on using such testing to avoid unnecessary major surgical procedures such as adrenalectomy. Unfortunately, the presence of estrogen receptors is not as specific for predicting favorable responses to ablative or hormone therapy as was initially hoped, 40-45 percent of patients with such receptors failing to improve, and 8 percent without such receptors improving after oophorectomy or adrenalectomy.[29]

With the use of suitable suppressive dosages of glucocorticoid, provided patients take them on an optimum schedule, it is possible that the beneficial effects of adrenalectomy in metastatic breast cancer might be obtained without submitting the patient to the major surgical procedure. This of course would not apply to ovariectomy, but this is a less strenuous surgical procedure. Furthermore, until our knowledge of the cause and treatment of cancer of the breast is more complete, the relative safety, plus the logic, of glucocorticoid therapy of this type would warrant its being tried in patients regardless of whether estrogen receptors were present in the tumor tissue.

The recent use of cytotoxic agents in the treatment of metastatic breast cancer has often included short courses of pharmacologic dosages of glucocorticoids, but it is possible that persistent administration of physiologic dosages of cortisone acetate or hydrocortisone might further improve the results of this type of therapy by persistently suppressing adrenal estrogen production.

Recently Santen and his associates have reported that aminoglutethimide, a chemical that blocks estrogen synthesis from androstenedione, lowers circulating and urinary levels of estrogen as well as adrenalectomy,[30] and they suggest that it may have value in the treatment of breast cancer. Because it also blocks conversion of cholesterol to pregnenolone, it inhibits cortisol production, and patients have to be given replacement hydrocortisone during its administration. This raises a question whether antitumor affects of aminoglutethimide would be greater than those of replacement dosages of hydrocortisone alone, provided such replacement dosages are administered on an optimum schedule for producing adrenal suppression. Replacement dosages of hydrocortisone should be less toxic.

It is also possible that physiologic dosages of cortisone or hydrocortisone might help patients with any type of malignancy by improving their resistance to the cancer. At present, two therapeutic principles seem important in the treatment of malignancy: the first is to destroy the malignant tissue, and cytotoxic drugs have produced impressive advances in this area. The second is to improve the resistance of the host. This principle has received less attention but may be equally important in the ultimate success of the therapy by impairing recurrences of tumor growth. Benjamini and Rennick[31] have recently summarized the present status of cancer immunotherapy, but glucocorticoids were not mentioned.

Treatment of patients with metastatic carcinoma of the prostate gland, where the tumor may be dependent upon androgen stimulation, has similar therapeutic possibilities. Historically, this was the first type of metastatic cancer that was reported to respond beneficially to adrenalectomy in patients who had had previous orchidectomy.

POSTOPERATIVE STATES

Another possible use of physiologic dosages of glucocorticoid is in certain postoperative states. When patients with adrenal insufficiency come to surgery, they are routinely given 100 mg of hydrocortisone sodium succinate (Solu-Cortef) intramuscularly one hour before surgery is begun; depending upon the illness of the patient and the extent of the surgical procedure, postoperatively they may receive 100 mg I.M. every eight hours for the first twenty-four hours, gradually tapering over the next week to their maintenance dose, or lower amounts down to 50 mg eight hours after the surgery followed by a resumption of usual maintenance dosage by mouth. Such patients have remarkably smooth postoperative courses, requiring little morphine or other pain-relieving medications, with restoration of strength, ambulation, and a good dietary intake sooner than many patients with normal adrenal function undergoing similar surgical procedures.

Beneficial effects of cortisone acetate in the postoperative state were reported very shortly after this steroid became available for clinical use,[32] but after harmful side effects with large doses were reported, possible beneficial effects of this type were apparently forgotten. Concerns regarding steroid administration in postoperative states, of course, are the possibility of interference with wound healing, increased susceptibility to infection, or possible masking of postoperative complications. During the past twenty-five years we have had sufficient experience with patients with adrenal insufficiency undergoing surgical procedures to indicate that dosages of hydrocortisone in the range that has been recommended will not cause any harmful effects. Wounds heal normally, and there is no indication of increased bacterial infection. None of these patients suffered complications of surgery, but experience with other patients who have required comparable doses at surgery due to previous glucocorticoid therapy indicates that such dosages do not mask surgical complications. Further studies of the potential value of this type of therapy in postoperative patients therefore seem warranted.

REFERENCES

1. Gibson M, Lackritz R, Schiff I, Tulchinsky D: Abnormal adrenal responses to adrenocorticotropic hormone in hyperandrogenic women. *Fertil Steril 33:*43-48, 1980.
2. Bardin CW, Lipsett MB: Testosterone and adrostenedione blood production rates in normal women and women with idiopathic hirsutism and polycystic ovaries. *J Clin Invest 46:*891-902, 1967.
3. Farber M, Millan VG, Turksoy RN, Mitchell GW, Jr.: Diagnostic evaluation of hirsutism in women by selective bilateral adrenal and ovarian venous catheterization. *Fertil Steril 30:*283-288, 1978.
4. Meikle AW, Stringham JD, Wilson DE, Dolman LI: Plasma 5α-reduced androgens in men and hirsute women: Role of adrenals and gonads. *J Clin Endocrinol Metab 48:*969-975, 1979.
5. Greenblatt RB, Mahesh VB: The androgenic polycystic ovary. *Am J Obstet Gynecol 125:*712-726, 1976.
6. Marx JL: Dysmenorrhea: Basic research leads to a rational therapy. *Science 205:*175-176, 1979.
7. Refetoff S, DeWind LT, DeGroot LJ: Familial syndrome combining deaf-mutism, stippled epiphyses, goiter and abnormally high PBI: Possible target organ refractoriness to thyroid hormone. *J Clin Endocrinol Metab 27:*279-294, 1967.
8. Refetoff S, DeGroot LJ, Bernard B, DeWind LT: Studies of a sibship with apparent hereditary resistance to the intracellular action of thyroid hormone. *Metabolism 21:*723-756, 1972.
9. Bernal J, Refetoff S, DeGroot LJ: Abnormalities of triiodothyronine binding to lymphocyte and fibroblast nuclei from a patient with peripheral resistance to thyroid hormone action. *J Clin Endocrinol Metab 47:*1266-1272, 1978.
10. Agerbaek H: Congenital goiter presumably resulting from tissue resistance to thyroid hormone. *Isr J Med Sci 8:*1859, 1970 (abstract).
11. Lamberg BA: Congenital euthyroid goiter and partial peripheral resistance to thyroid hormones. *Lancet 1:*854-857, 1973.
12. Bode HH, Danon M, Weintraub BD, Maloof F, Crawford JD: Partial target organ resistance to thyroid hormone. *J Clin Invest 52:*776-782, 1973.
13. Schneider G, Keiser HR, Bardin CW: Peripheral resistance to thyroxine: a cause for short stature in a boy without goiter. *Clin Endocrinol (Oxf) 4:*111-118, 1975.

14. Lamberg BA, Sandström R, Rosengord S, Saarinen P, Evered DC: Sporadic and familial partial peripheral resistance to thyroid hormone. In Harland WA, Orr JS (Eds.): *Thyroid Hormone Metabolism.* London, Acad Pr, 1975, pp 139-161.

15. Elewaut A, Mussche M, Vermeulen A: Familial partial target organ resistance to thyroid hormone. *J Clin Endocrinol Metab 43:*575-581, 1976.

16. Hill SR, Jr., Reiss RS, Forsham PH, Thorn GW: The effect of adrenocorticotropin and cortisone on thyroid function: Thyroid-adrenocortical interrelationships. *J Clin Endocrinol 10:*1375-1400, 1950.

17. Beierwaltes WH, Wolfson WQ, Jones JR, Knorpp CT, Siemienski JS: Increase in basal oxygen consumption produced by cortisone in patients with untreated myxedema. (Abst.) *J Lab Clin Med 36:*799, 1950.

18. Werner SC, Hamilton H, Frantz VK: Some effects of ACTH in chronic thyroiditis and myxedema. In Mote J (Ed.): *Proceedings of Second Clinical ACTH Conference,* Vol. 2. Philadelphia, Blakiston, 1951, pp 521-528.

19. Lerman J, Harington CR, Means JH: Physiologic activity of some analogues of thyroxine. *J Clin Endocrinol Metab 12:*1306-1314, 1952.

20. Thorn GW, Jenkins D, Laidlaw JC, Goetz FC, Dingman JF, Arons WL, Streeten DHP, McCracken BH: Pharmacologic aspects of adrenocortical steroids and ACTH in man. *N Engl J Med 248:*232-245, 284-294, 323-337, 369-378, 414-423, 588-601, 632-646, 1953.

21. Jefferies WMcK: Effect of physiologic dosages of cortisone on circulating T3: apparent correction of partial peripheral resistance to T3 and improvement in conversion of T4 to T3. Unpublished paper.

22. Chopra IJ, Williams DE, Orgiazzi J, Solomon DH: Opposite effects of dexamethasone on serum concentrations of 3, 3',5' triiodothyronine (reverse T3) and 3, 3',5 triiodothyronine (T3). *J Clin Endocrinol Metab 41:*911-916, 1975.

23. Bermudez F, Surks MI, Oppenheimer JH: High incidence of decreased serum triiodothyronine concentration in patients with non-thyroidal disease. *J Clin Endocrinol Metab 41:*27-40, 1975.

24. Johnson DD, Dorr KE, Swenson WM, Service FJ: Reactive hypoglycemia. *JAMA 243:*1151-1155, 1980.

25. Altschule MD, Promisel E, Parkhurst BH, Grunebaum H: Effects of ACTH in patients with mental diseases. *Arch Neurol Psychiatry 64:*641-649, 1950.

26. Elithorn A, Bridges PK, Hodges JR: Adrenocortical responsiveness during courses of electroconvulsive therapy. *Br J Psychiatry 115:*575-580, 1969.

27. Ingle DJ: The role of the adrenal cortex in homeostasis. *J Clin Endocrinol 8:*23-27, 1952.

28. Granner DK: The role of glucocorticoid hormones as biologic amplifiers. In Baxter JD, Rousseau GG (Eds.): *Glucocorticoid Hormone Action.* New York, Springer-Verlag, 1979, pp 593-611.

29. Henderson IC, Canellos GP: Cancer of the breast: The past decade. *N Engl J Med 302:*78-90, 1980.

30. Samojzik E, Veldhuis JD, Wells SA, Santen RJ: Preservation of androgen secretion during estrogen suppression with aminoglutethimide in the treatment of metastatic breast carcinoma. *J Clin Invest 65:*602-612, 1980.

31. Benjamini E, Rennick DM: Cancer Immunotherapy: Facts and Fancy. *CA – A Cancer Journal for Clinicians 29:*362-370, 1979.

32. Hume DM, Moore FD: The use of ACTH, cortisone and adrenal cortical extracts in surgical patients. In Mote JR (Ed.): *Proceedings of Second Clinical ACTH Conference,* Vol 2. Philadelphia, Blakiston, 1951, pp 289-309.

Chapter 11

SUMMARY AND SPECULATION

THESE OBSERVATIONS, spanning thirty years of experience with glucocorticoid therapy, obviously raise more questions than they answer. As a clinical investigator with limited research facilities I have not been able to do more than scratch the surface of the potential of this type of treatment, but I hope the previous chapters have convinced the reader that cortisone or hydrocortisone therapy can be safe and that the potential of safe glucocorticoid therapy is sufficiently great to warrant further study.

In conclusion, I would like to indulge in some speculation regarding a few of the possibilities raised in the preceding chapters. Although a few of these suggestions may seem rather remote and tenuous, they are based on logic and may provide a stimulus for future studies.

If the adrenal cortex does produce an anti-sodium-retaining factor as postulated in Chapter 3, it is possible that some cases of hypertension may result from a deficiency of this factor. Such cases would probably have low levels of renin because of the relative excess of sodium-retaining hormone, but the actual levels of this hormone would not be elevated. The possible sequence of events in the development of hypertension in such cases might be as follows: (1) a deficient intake of water relative to salt, producing an increased requirement for anti-sodium-retaining factor; (2) with prolonged maintenance of such a state, the ability to produce anti-sodium-retaining factor might become deficient or exhausted; (3) excessive sodium retention and hypertension would then result. The possibility that a relative deficiency of water intake might contribute to the production of hypertension should therefore be studied, as well as the possibility that an increased intake of water in addition to a decreased intake of sodium might be beneficial in the treatment of hypertension, provided the steroid abnormality or renal damage has not become irreversible.

The phenomenon of low adrenal reserve needs to be further investigated, both with regard to its definition and its relation to conditions such as allergies, autoimmune disorders, postviral syndrome, and chronic fatigue. Why it seems to be temporary in some instances and permanent in others also needs clarification.

The role of glucocorticoids in the immune process obviously is a challenge for further research. Why and how physiologic dosages enhance immunity whereas pharmacologic dosages reduce resistance must be determined. Whether the apparent enhancement of circulating levels of immune globulins, especially IgM, by physiologic dosages is a significant factor in the improvement of immunity must be answered, as well as whether effects on other aspects of the immune response may contribute.

The possible contribution of other adrenal hormones to immunity should also be investigated. An observation made fifteen years ago on a thirty year old woman taking dehydroepiandrosterone (DHA) suggests that this adrenal androgen may affect resistance to infection. This patient had irregular menses and a fertility problem, and fractionation of urinary 17-ketosteroids revealed an absence of DHA. Because a supply of this steroid was available for clinical investigation, she was given 5 mg daily by mouth for six weeks, then 5 mg twice daily for a month, then three times daily for a month, then four times daily. She had both subjective and objective improvement on the first three dosages, but two weeks after increasing to 5 mg four times daily, she developed an upper respiratory infection complicated by herpes simplex, a condition she had not previously experienced, suggesting that the larger dosage may have caused some decrease in resistance. Fractionation of urinary 17-KS was performed while she was on each dosage, and after the dosage was increased to 5 mg four times daily, urinary 11-oxygenated 17-KS dropped to zero and remained zero until the dosage was reduced, suggesting that the larger dosage of DHA had interfered with 11-beta-hydroxylation. Unfortunately, our limited supply of DHA did not permit further studies of this question.

The coincidence of apparent decrease in resistance at the time when 11-beta-hydroxylation was reduced suggested a relationship, however. Since 11-beta-hydroxylation is the last enzymatic step in the pathway of production of hydrocortisone, it is tempting to speculate that the apparent decrease in resistance may have been due to a decreased ability to produce hydrocortisone. A reduction in dosage to 5 mg once or twice daily seemed to provide optimum benefit. Although the apparent effect upon resistance could be coincidental, the possibility that smaller dosages of DHA may benefit resistance and larger dosages decrease it should be studied further. Also the possibility that larger dosages of DHA may impair production of hydrocortisone through decreasing 11-beta-hydroxylation needs confirmation.

Studies of the relationship of adrenocortical hormones to immunity should include not only the processes involved in resistance to infections of all types, viral, fungal, bacterial, rickettsial, and protozoal, but also those involved in resistance to malignancy. We need to start studying factors involved in protection of the body from the development and growth of malignant cells as well as to continue to study means of destroying malignant cells.

The relationship of adrenocortical response to infection must be related to the response to other stresses. For example, evidence suggests that as an initial response to stress increased utilization of hydrocortisone occurs. This, plus the increased need for hydrocortisone to combat the stress, results in symptoms and changes in blood chemistry consistent with relative adrenal insufficiency during the shock phase of the alarm reaction. The adrenals then apparently respond with increased production of hydrocortisone as a result of stimulation by ACTH. Because there is increased utilization of hydrocortisone, plasma cortisol levels may not increase very much, but a drop in circulating eosinophils reflects the increased glucocorticoid effect. Leukocytosis with an increase in granulocytes and decrease in lymphocytes is also characteristic of glucocorticoid effect. Such changes occur with bacterial infections, but the lack of leukocytosis, granulocytosis, lymphopenia, or eosinopenia in viral infections suggests an absence of normal adrenocortical response, and our observation of low plasma cortisol levels during the early phase of influenza is consistent with this possibility, but other factors may also contribute to these differences. The adrenal response to stress therefore appears to be an important component of the body's nonspecific mechanism of resistance to infection, and if it is sufficient, the host may not develop any clinical symptoms of illness.

If this speculation is correct, the nonspecific symptoms of illness, such as malaise, anorexia, and fatigue, may be manifestations of relative adrenal insufficiency and may not be a necessary component of the body's defense mechanism at all. Consistent with this possibility is the observation that some patients taking cortisone acetate or hydrocortisone, 5 mg four times daily, upon developing symptoms of an incipient upper respiratory infection and doubling their dosage of steroid, experienced a complete clearing of symptoms, suggesting that the infection had been aborted. Others on the same treatment continued to develop symptoms of the illness, suggesting either that they had a more virulent infection or that their basal resistance was lower and, hence, not raised sufficiently to prevent the illness. If the latter is correct, increasing the dosage of steroid by three- or four-fold might be more effective in aborting the illness. Studies of persons who report they never had common respiratory illnesses to determine how their immune response differs from that of people who are subject to such infections would be of interest. Also studies of differences in the state of the immune mechanism during the spring and autumn, the seasons of greatest incidence of respiratory illnesses in temperate climates, compared with summer and winter might be helpful.

Factors determining whether large dosages of glucocorticoids enhance or impair immunity must be clarified. Both the timing of administration relative to the onset of infection and the size of the dosage seem important. If hydrocortisone or other glucocorticoids are administered in sufficient dosage to suppress the hypothalamic-pituitary-adrenal response *prior to* exposure to infection or toxin, resistance may be lowered or possibly distorted, whereas comparable large doses, perhaps provided they are not too large, administered *after* exposure to infections or toxins may improve resistance. The studies of Thomas and Good,[1] which demonstrated that the Schwartzman phenomenon of hemorrhagic necrosis at the site of injection of toxin occurred when large doses of cortisone were administered prior to, but not when they were administered after, the injection of toxin, are consistent with this clinical impression. Because the Schwartzman phenomenon is apparently a type of autoimmune reaction, these studies also suggest that autoimmune disorders may be related to an impairment of the immune process prior to the onset of a stress such as an infection or exposure to toxin.

Observations of Kass and Finland made shortly after cortisone was introduced[2] indicate that the *size* of glucocorticoid dosage also may be a determining factor in response to infections. They noted that the amount of cortisone required to restore adrenalectomized mice to approximately the original state of resistance to infection was five to ten times the amount that maintained uninfected adrenalectomized mice in an apparently normal state, whereas approximately twenty to fifty times the minimum maintenance dosage must be given to depress the mouse's resistance below that of an intact animal. In our clinical observations, the ratios are not so great, a mere doubling of the maintenance dosage often apparently being sufficient to protect against common respiratory infections, and an excess of glucocorticoid much less than the twenty-to fiftyfold increase necessary to reduce resistance in the adrenalectomized mouse may be sufficient to impair resistance in the human.

The evidence that factors that are known to lower resistance to infection, such as lack of sleep, poor nutrition, and excessive fatigue, also increase the strain on the adrenal cortex is consistent with the importance of this gland in protecting against disease. That some persons never have common respiratory illnesses suggests that there is a great difference in individual innate resistance, at least to some viral infections. The characteristic lowering of resistance to bacterial infections following viral infections may be related to an inhibition or distortion of the hypothalamic-pituitary-adrenal mechanism by the viral infection or by depletion of glucocorticoids in response to the infection. Conversely, increased resistance to other stresses that occurs during the stage of resistance of the general adaptation syndrome may be at least partly due to a state of increased adrenocortical activity.

After the initial "shock" response to acute stress or infection the countershock phase occurs, characterized by evidence of increased production of hydrocortisone, and when this response, plus any specific immune response such as increased production of antibodies, is sufficient, the infection is overcome and the patient recovers. If the subject's resistance is lowered due to chronic debility, poor nutrition, inadequate rest, previous stress, or infection, the immune response, including production of hydrocortisone, may be impaired, and the symptoms and duration of the illness may be greater. In some circumstances, the infection itself, as in certain virus infections, may interfere with normal hypothalamic-pituitary-adrenal response, and the patient may succumb rapidly either to the initial infection or to some complicating infection as a result of interference with normal host defenses. In such cases, the administration of proper additional dosages of cortisone acetate or hydrocortisone may be beneficial in overcoming the infection more quickly or may even be lifesaving. It is essential that other supportive therapy and, in the presence of bacterial infections, suitable antibiotics be administered concomitantly with the steroid.

When such a program of therapy is initiated, it appears to be advisable to continue it until the patient is completely recovered and feeling well. This certainly applies to antibiotic therapy, which must be continued for several days after the patient has apparently recovered so as to minimize the chance of recurrence. The increased dosage of cortisone acetate or hydrocortisone should also be continued until the patient is feeling well, then tapered to the pre-illness maintenance level within a few days, or in patients who have not previously been receiving glucocorticoid therapy, tapered and withdrawn completely. This contrasts with the usual recommendations for decreasing glucocorticoid dosages more slowly after a maximum therapeutic response of larger doses has been achieved in conditions such as collagen disorders. There is no indication that this therapy of infections causes any problems; on the contrary, it seems to shorten the duration and severity of clinical symptoms and decrease the incidence of complications.

The mechanism by which glucocorticoids increase resistance needs further investigation. Additional studies of the effects of physiologic as well as pharmacologic dosages of glucocorticoids upon immune globulins are needed, and because of the apparent important role of interferon in the immune response[3] plus the similarity of some of its effects to those of physiologic dosages of glucocorticoids, the effect of glucocorticoid upon interferon production and activity should be investigated. Because of proven importance of the complement system in defense against microbial infection, especially the contribution of properdin and the alternative pathway of complement activation to natural, nonimmune defense as well as to amplifying antibody-dependent reactions[4] the effect of varying dosages of glucocorticoids on this system should be studied.

The factors affecting the resting levels and responses to stress of plasma cortisol and possibly other adrenal cortical steroids such as DHA need further study. The significance of the diurnal pattern of production of these hormones must be determined. It is known that when subreplacement dosages of cortisone acetate or hydrocortisone are administered, ACTH is secreted in its usual diurnal pattern, but in smaller amounts. This may explain part of the beneficial effect of subreplacement dosages of cortisone or hydrocortisone, but more information is needed regarding factors that affect ACTH stimulation or suppression. Because "ectopic" secretory episodes of cortisol occur most frequently between the sixth and eighth hours of sleep and the fewest episodes two to four hours prior to the onset of sleep, it appears that adequate sleep increases sensitivity of the hypothalamic-pituitary-adrenal mechanism with increased production of ACTH and plasma cortisol, whereas fatigue produces a converse effect. Nutrition also probably affects the function of the hypothalamic-pituitary-adrenal axis, and intake and utilization of vitamin C seem especially likely to affect the efficiency of this axis. Hence, a clarification of the possible relationship between ascorbic acid metabolism and adrenocortical function is needed. The evidence that patients with allergies frequently have low baseline levels of plasma cortisol should be confirmed, and the reasons why some persons have relatively low or relatively high resting levels of this or other steroids would be of interest.

Studies of the role of leukocytes in the immune response in recent years have provided fascinating insight into the actions of these cells. It is evident that thymus-derived or T-lymphocytes provide the nonspecific, cellular response to infection, and B-lymphocytes provide specific antibodies. The T-lymphocytes can be further divided into helper T-cells, which assist the immune response, including the production of antibody by B-cells, and suppressor T-cells, which regulate and shut off the immune response when it has achieved its purpose. Because a deficiency of suppressor T-cells appears to be responsible for the development of at least some autoimmune disorders, wherein the body develops antibodies to some of its own tissues or immune complexes that interfere with normal functions, and because hydrocortisone suppresses autoimmune disorders, it is possible that hydrocortisone stimulates suppressor cell activity under at least some circumstances. Excessive suppressor cell activity might be a mechanism by which excessive dosages of glucocorticoids impair resistance. Hence, studies of the effects of physiologic versus pharmacologic levels of hydrocortisone upon T-cell activity should be interesting.

The mechanism of improvement in energy and feeling of well-being that occurs in some persons while taking subreplacement dosages of cortisone or hydrocortisone needs further study. This seems to be different from the euphoria that may occur with pharmacologic dosages of glucocorticoids in that it is not associated with any tendency to psychosis, and it may persist for long periods of time after withdrawal of the glucocorticoid in contrast to the relatively rapid loss of the euphoria after the discontinuance of pharmacologic dosages. The evidence that subreplacement dosages may correct a partial receptor block for triiodothyronine plus the evidence that high normal circulating levels of T_3 by RIA decrease during the administration of subreplacement dosages suggests that an improvement in receptor function for triiodothyronine may be a mechanism underlying the apparent nonspecific improvement in energy that occurs with this dosage. It is also evident that an improvement in energy occurs in patients with allergic disorders when they receive subreplacement dosages, so the effect of this therapy upon cellular receptors for triiodothyronine in patients with the "immediate type" hypersensitivity disorders would be of interest.

It has been demonstrated that the active form of thyroid hormone is T_3 and that T_3 acts within the nuclei of cells. Hence, T_3 must move from the blood stream, where it is circulating, to the cell nucleus, where it combines with receptors and produces an increase in metabolism. Because T_3 is a protein, it cannot cross cell membranes without help, but the nature of this helper is not known. The ultimate action of thyroid hormone could therefore depend upon the efficiency of this helper as well as upon other critical steps in its utilization. Because hydrocortisone appears to improve the utilization of T_3 in patients with symptoms of hypothyroidism and elevated T_3 by RIA, and because it seems to cause a decrease in circulating T_3 by RIA when this is in upper normal range, it seems likely that hydrocortisone, at least under some circumstances, improves the function of this helper or of the T_3 receptor.

In hypothyroidism, on the other hand, hydrocortisone does not cause a decrease in circulating T_3 by RIA but rather tends to produce an increase. This observation, plus the decrease in circulating T_4 that often occurs simultaneously, and the improvement in energy manifested in such patients, suggests that the hydrocortisone is enhancing conversion of T_4 to T_3. Thus physiologic dosages of hydrocortisone appear to be capable of improving thyroid hormone activity by increasing conversion of T_4 to T_3 as well as by enhancing T_3 effect on the cell.

In hypothyroidism, an increase in T_3 receptors would be expected, so the failure to produce a decrease in circulating T_3 suggests that the effect of hydrocortisone on receptor function may depend on the number of T_3 receptors. Hence, if the number of T_3 receptors is high, but the amount of T_3 is low, as in hypothyroidism, hydrocortisone has little or no effect; if the number of T_3 receptors and level of circulating T_3 is normal, it improves receptor function. If the number of unoccupied T_3 receptors is low, as in hyperthyroidism, clinical experience suggests that T_3 receptor activity is also increased by hydrocortisone. The patient in Case 8 of Chapter 4, a man with congenital adrenal hyperplasia who had a recurrence of hyperthyroidism after treatment with hydrocortisone, 5 mg four times daily, seems to support this speculation. If this is true, administration of small dosages of glucocorticoid to patients with untreated Graves' disease might cause an increase in hypermetabolism, but administration with antithyroid therapy does not seem to produce this effect. The observation, referred to in Chapter 8, of Hill and his associates[5] that the administratoin of ACTH or cortisone to patients with Graves' disease seemed to produce a transient exacerbation followed by a decrease in thyroid function suggests that larger dosages may counteract the underlying cause of this disorder and is consistent with the beneficial effect of glucocorticoids in autoimmune diseases.

If the number of receptors is high and the amount of circulating thyroid hormone is high, as in pregnancy, the administration of a small dosage of hydrocortisone may improve receptor activity, and this may be a mechanism of its apparent protection against miscarriage. This may explain why the administration of small dosages of hydrocortisone or of additional thyroid hormone seem to protect against miscarriage in women prone to this problem. The increased receptor activity could increase the effectiveness of thyroid hormone already present, whereas the administration of additional thyroid hormone would be another means of providing increased thyroid effect. Yet, this would not explain why some patients seem to require both additional thyroid and a small dosage of cortisone or hydrocortisone to protect their pregnancies, whereas others seem to require only one or the other. Perhaps cortisone or hydrocortisone may improve estrogen receptor function also, and this may be a mechanism of some of their beneficial effects in patients with ovarian dysfunction as well as in habitual aborters.

Finally, although much has been learned regarding the components of energy metabolism and of the immune response, little is known of the mechanisms regulating these vital processes. Circumstantial evidence suggests a significant role of physiologic amounts of hydrocortisone in such regulation, so it is therefore time to discard the indiscriminate fear that has resulted from the harmful side effects of excessive dosages of glucocorticoids and return to the study of the role of physiologic amounts of the natural glucocorticoids in maintaining health and energy, and of the potential of safe, physiologic dosages of these steroids in improving the body's overall resistance to infection, malignancy, and other stresses.

REFERENCES

1. Thomas L, Good RA: The effect of cortisone on the Schwartzman reaction. *J Exp Med 95:*409-428, 1952.
2. Kass E, Finland M: Adrenocortical hormones in infection and immunity. *Ann Rev Microbiol 7:*361-388, 1953, p 368.
3. Marks JWL: Interferon: (I) On the threshold of clinical application. *Science 204:*1185-1186, 1979.
4. Fearon DT, Austin KF: The alternative pathway of complement — A system for host resistance to microbial infection. *N Engl J Med 303:*259-263, 1980.
5. Hill SR Jr., Reiss RS, Forsham PH, Thorn GW: The effect of adrenocorticotropin and cortisone on thyroid function: Thyroid-adrenocortical interrelationships. *J Clin Endocrinol 10:*1375-1400, 1950.

PROPRIETARY TRADE NAMES
FOR PHARMACEUTICALS
MENTIONED IN TEXT

Acthar-gel — corticotropin

Armour Pharmaceutical Company
6991 East Camelback Rd. Suite
  A-210
Scottsdale, Arizona 85251

Aldomet — methyldopa

Merck, Sharp & Dohme
West Point, Pennsylvania 19486

Aristocort — triamcinolone

Lederle Laboratories
Wayne, N.J. 07470

Bellergal — contains phenobarbital,
  20 mg, ergotamine tartrate, 0.3
  mg, and belladonna, 0.1 mg

Dorsey Laboratories
P.O. Box 83288
Lincoln, Nebraska 68501

Cortef — hydrocortisone

The Upjohn Company
7000 Portage Road
Kalamazoo, Michigan 49001

Cortrosyn — active ACTH fraction

Organon, Inc.
375 Mt. Pleasant Avenue
West Orange, N.J. 07052

Cytomel — liothyronine sodium

Smith, Kline & French
P.O. Box 7929
Philadelphia, Pennsylvania 19101

Dilantin — sodium phenytoin

Parke-Davis & Company
201 Tabor Road
Morris Plains, N.J. 07950

Diuril — chlorothiazide

Merck, Sharp & Dohme
West Point, Pennsylvania 19486

Elavil — amitriptyline HCl

Merck, Sharp & Dohme
West Point, Pennsylvania 19486

Euthroid — sodium l-thyroxine and
  sodium liothyronine in 4:1 ratio

Parke-Davis & Company
201 Tabor Road
Morris Plains, N.J. 07950

181

Florinef — fludrocortisone acetate	Squibb & Sons, Inc. P.O. Box 4000 Princeton, N.J. 08540
Halotestin — fluoxymestrone	The Upjohn Company 7000 Portage Road Kalamazoo, Michigan 49001
Hydrodiuril — hydrochlorothiazide	Merck, Sharp & Dohme West Point, Pennsylvania 19486
Inderal — propranolol hydrochloride	Ayerst Laboratories 685 Third Avenue New York, NY 10017
Marax — ephedrine sulfate, theophylline, hydroxyzine HCl	Roerig 235 East 42nd Street New York, NY 10017
Metopirone — metyrapone	Ciba Pharmaceutical Co. Summit, N.J. 07901
Motrin — ibuprofen	The Upjohn Company 7000 Portage Road Kalamazoo, Michigan 49001
Multicebrin — pan-vitamins	Eli Lilly and Co. 307 E. McCarty Street Indianapolis, Indiana 46285
Plaquenil Sulfate — hydroxy-chloroquine sulfate	Winthrop Laboratories 90 Park Avenue New York, N.Y. 10016
Premarin — conjugated estrogens	Ayerst Laboratories 685 Third Avenue New York, N.Y. 10017
Pro-Banthine — propantheline bromide	Searle Laboratories Box 5110 Chicago, Illinois 60680
Provera — medroxyprogesterone acetate	The Upjohn Company 7000 Portage Road Kalamazoo, Michigan 49001
Quadrinal — ephedrine HCl, phenobarbital, theophylline calcium salicylate and potassium iodide	Knoll Pharmaceutical Company 30 North Jefferson Road Whippany, N.J. 07981
Solu-Cortef — hydrocortisone sodium succinate	The Upjohn Company 7000 Portage Road Kalamazoo, Michigan 49001

Synthroid — sodium levothyroxine

Flint Laboratories
Deerfield, Illinois 60015

Tapazole — methimazole

Eli Lilly and Company
307 E. McCarty Street
Indianapolis, Indiana 46285

Thorazine — chlorpromazine

Smith, Kline and French
P.O. Box 7929
Philadelphia, Pennsylvania 19101

Valium — diazepan

Roche Laboratories
Nutley, N.J. 07110

NORMAL VALUES FOR TESTS LISTED
IN CASE SUMMARIES

Urine

17-ketosteroids	5-15 mg/24 hr
17-hydroxycorticosteroids (Porter-Silber)	5-11 mg/24 hr
Cortisol metabolites (Michelakis)	7-17 mg/24 hr
FSH (follicle-stimulating hormone)	8-32 mouse uterine units/24 hours
Total estrogens	4-60 mcg/24 hr

Blood

erythrocyte sedimentation rate	0-20 mm/hr (female)
serum PBI (protein-bound iodine)	3.8-8.0 mcg/dl
serum cholesterol	150-260 mg/dl
T_3 sponge uptake	40-60%
T_4	4.5-10.0 mcg/dl
T_3 index	0.8-1.2
T_3 by RIA (radioimmunoassay)	65-215 ng/dl
plasma FSH (follicle-stimulating hormone)	
female — pre-ovulatory	15-30 mIU/ml
male	5-40 mIU/ml
plasma ACTH by RIA	15-100 pg/ml
plasma cortisol by RIA	
8 AM	15-25 mcg/dl
5 PM	5-10 mcg/dl
plasma desoxycorticosterone	5-15 ng/dl
plasma total estrogens	
female — pre-ovulatory	45-200 pg/ml
male	10-80 pg/ml
plasma estradiol —	
female — preovulatory	15-75 pg/ml
plasma testosterone	
female	0.0-0.1 mcg/dl

Miscellaneous

I^{131} uptake (thyroid)	15-30% in 24 hr

NAME INDEX

A

Adams, C. H., 11
Addison, Thomas, 36
Adelson, L., 144
Agerbaek, H., 166
Albert, A., 11, 25
Albright, Fuller, vii-ix, xi, 25
Alexander, J., xi, 25
Alpert, Elmer, viii
Altschule, M. D., 65, 167
Ambrose, C. T., 127, 143
Anderson, T. W., 143
Andrews, R. V., 53, 65, 69, 91
Arons, W. L., 11, 167
Aschoff, L., 125, 142
Atherdem, S. M., 65
Austin, K. F., 179

B

Bach, F., 103
Bader, M. E., 26
Baker, B. L., 12, 25
Barbato, A. L., 26
Bardin, C. W., 166
Barker, M. W., 15, 26
Barnes, E. W., 65
Barnes, N. D., 65
Barnes, P., 109
Bartter, Frederick C., viii, xi, 25
Baxter, J. D., 167
Beaton, G. H., 143
Beck, J. C., 25
Beierwaltes, W. H., 122, 154, 167
Beisel, W. R., 35, 125, 127, 142
Bellet, S., 65
Benacerraf, B., 108
Bender, C. E., 139, 144

Benedek, T. G., 126, 143
Benjamini, E., 164, 168
Bennett, L. L., 25
Berger, S., 142, 144
Bermudez, F., 167
Bernal, J., 166
Bernard, B., 166
Blades, R., 144
Blanchard, E. W., 128, 143
Bode, H. H., 166
Boland, E. W., 100, 103
Bonner, C. D., 102
Bonomo, I., 11
Borkin, R. E., 103
Bosworth, D. C., 142
Boyle, J. A., 65
Bridges, P. K., 65, 167
Briot, M., 108
Brown, J., 111, 122
Brown, M., 109
Browning, McK., 65
Bunim, J. J., 103
Burston, R. A., 26

C

Canary, J. H., 35
Canellos, G. P., 168
Caplan, R. M., 92
Carreon, G., 35
Carroll, E., xi, 25
Chappel, M. R., 139, 144
Chase, J. H., 129, 143
Chopra, I. J., 167
Claxton, H. E., 11
Clayton, B. E., 65
Clerkin, E., 35
Coburn, J. W., 122
Cohen, A., 103
Colby, H. D., 91
Conn, J. W., 25
Coombs, R. R. A., 65, 104, 108

Cooper, G., 26, 65
Cope, C. L., 30, 35
Corcoran, A. C., 25
Coyne, M. D., 91
Craighead, J. E., 123
Crawford, J. D., 166
Cristofafnini, A., 144
Crohn, B., 121, 123
Cruz-Coke, R., 144
Crymble, M., 25

D

Dailey, M. P., 102
Daniels, C. A., 144
Danon, M., 166
DeAndrade, J. R., 26, 103
DeCastro, O., 65
DeGroot, L. J., 154, 166
Dempsey, E. L., xi, 25
Dempsey, H., 94, 101-102
DeWind, L. T., 154, 166
Dias-Rivera, R., 144
Diercks, F. H., 144
Dingman, J. F., 11, 167
Dluhy, R. G., 66
Dobriner, K., 35
Dollery, C., 109
Dolman, L. I., 166
Dorfman, R. J., 66
Dorr, K. E., 167
Dougherty, T. F., 129, 143
Douglas, A. C., 144
Dowling, J. T., 122
Duff, I. F., 122
Dunkelman, S. S., 35
Dustan, H. P., 25
Dwyer, J. M., 144

E

Ebert, R. V., 27
Einhorn, J., 111, 122
Elewaut, A., 167

185

SUBJECT INDEX